What Language Does Your Patient Hurt In?

A Practical Guide to Culturally Competent Patient Care

SECOND EDITION

Suzanne Salimbene
Diversity Resources, Inc. Amherst, MA

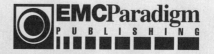

Developmental Editor: Courtney Kost
Proofreader: Susan Capecchi
Cover Designer: C. Vern Johnson
Desktop Production Specialist: Petrina Nyhan
Text Designer: Jennifer Wreisner

Acknowledgements
The publisher, author, and editor would like to thank Jan Jenner, Ph.D., of Rendalia Biologists, Talladega, Alabama, for her valuable contributions to this text.

Diversity Resources, Inc.™, Amherst, MA 01002 © 2000, 2005 by Suzanne Salimbene
All rights reserved. First edition 2000 Second edition 2005 Printed in the United States of America
Republished by Paradigm Publishing Inc. with permission of Diversity Resources™.

Published by **EMC**Paradigm
875 Montreal Way
St. Paul, MN 55102

(800) 535-6865
E-mail: educate@emcp.com
Web site: www.emcp.com

Care has been taken to provide accurate and useful information about the Internet and specific Web sites. However, the author, editor, and publisher cannot accept any responsibility for Web, e-mail, newsgroup, or chatroom subject matter nor content, nor for consequences from any application of the information in this book, and make no warranty, expressed or implied, with respect to the book's content.

Text: ISBN 0-7638-2333-3
Product Number 01678

Printed in the United States of America.

10 9 8 7 6 5 4 3

Contents

CHAPTER 4. PROVIDING CULTURE-SENSITIVE HEALTH CARE TO PATIENTS OF ASIAN ORIGIN   31

CHAPTER 5. PROVIDING CULTURE-SENSITIVE HEALTH CARE TO HISPANIC/LATINO PATIENTS   43

CHAPTER 6. PROVIDING CULTURE-SENSITIVE HEALTH CARE TO PEOPLE FROM THE MIDDLE EAST   51

CHAPTER 7. PROVIDING CULTURE-SENSITIVE HEALTH CARE TO EMIGRÉS FROM THE FORMER SOVIET BLOC COUNTRIES OF RUSSIA, BOSNIA, AND POLAND

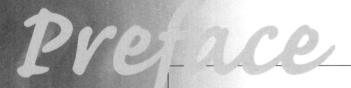

Preface

When this guide was first published, the issue of culturally competent patient care was just emerging as a concern within the healthcare community. Since then, with the steady growth of Hispanic and other ethnic and racial groups in proportion to the total population, the question of how to provide a high level of quality healthcare to these groups has moved to the center of the national healthcare agenda. Once considered primarily an issue of providing interpreters who could bridge the linguistic gap between English-speaking providers and non-English-speaking patients, culturally competent patient care is now recognized by the health community as having as much, if not more, to do with cultural understanding as it does with interpretation of medical information.

With the publication of its final report on *National Standards for Culturally and Linguistically Appropriate Services in Health Care* (CLAS) in March 2001, the Department of Health and Human Services Office of Minority Health heralded this new era in healthcare. Cultural and linguistic sensitivity, awareness, and knowledge were now defined as an intrinsic element in a healthcare provider's ability to provide quality medical care and services. Other government offices such as the Office for Civil Rights (OCR), the Centers for Medicare and Medicaid Services (CMS), and the Health Resources and Services Administration (HRSA) soon followed with their own efforts to ensure that quality care is accessible and appropriate to the linguistic and cultural needs of all minority populations.

The Joint Commission on Accreditation of Healthcare Organizations (JCAHO) is also engaged in a major research project funded by the California Endowment to assess the ability of hospitals to address the issues of language and culture that affect the quality and safety of patient care. The attention now given by governmental and accreditation agencies to eliminating disparities in access to quality healthcare due to language and cultural differences has made the development of cultural and linguistic competence necessary for the very survival of individual practitioners as well as healthcare institutions. While more and more medical and nursing schools are adding at least some training in cultural and linguistic competence to their curricula, and a number of such programs in continuing medical education and nursing education are coming onto the market, medical and nursing staff already working in the field are most often left to develop these skills on their own.

This guide provides an efficient and practical means by which cultural and linguistic competence can be achieved either inside or outside the classroom.

The general format is the same as in the first edition. The information and references have been updated to include much of the new and exciting work that has been done in this field since the publication of the first edition. I have also tried to respond to questions and requests from readers.

The introduction includes an expanded section on avoiding stereotypes that provides a series of questions to ask patients in order to develop a profile of individual health, illness, and illness prevention beliefs and practices. These questions are also designed to assist in the assessment of the patient's degree of assimilation into mainstream American culture and/or his or her degree of adherence to the traditional health practices and beliefs of the cultural group to which the patient is assumed to belong. The patient's answers to these questions can then be used to negotiate a treatment plan that is in accord with the patient's belief system and meets his or her cultural needs and expectations. A treatment plan that takes these beliefs into consideration will not only lead to greater patient compliance with the plan but also enhance the patient's trust for the caregiver and the healthcare system as a whole.

Chapter 1 includes an expanded section on tips for improving the cross-cultural relationship between the caregiver and the patient, as well as two new sections on tips for determining the individual etiquette, beliefs, and practices of patients from other cultures and tips for assessing and counseling patients on diet and nutrition. A new section on the health beliefs and practices of Hmong refugees has been added to chapter 4. Chapter 8 is an entirely new chapter that discusses the possible effects of certain religious beliefs on health/illness practices. This chapter includes information on the religious beliefs of the Amish, Christian Scientists, Eastern Orthodox Christians, Jehovah's Witnesses, Jews, and Mormons, as well as a set of tips for offering care to diverse religious groups. While religious groups are not necessarily culturally diverse, differences in religious laws and in perspectives on health maintenance and cures can seriously affect response to and compliance with medical care and services.

Each of the other chapters contains new material incorporating research conducted since the publication of the first edition as well as a more detailed treatment of each cultural group that is discussed.

To busy caregivers who have all they can do to keep up with the current literature in their field, the new requirements of cultural and linguistic competency may seem an insurmountable burden. I hope that this guide will help to ease this burden and provide the information required in an easily accessible format.

How to Use the Guide

The guide contains a brief summary of the health/illness/illness prevention beliefs and practices as well as the religious beliefs and taboos of the major cultural groups living in the United States. It suggests effective ways to develop successful relationships with patients from each group. This knowledge is essential to effective patient care. However, although the cultural information provided in the guide is a viable starting point, it is essential to question each patient individually to determine his or her degree of assimilation into U.S. culture and the healthcare system.

Although members of our caregiving community are trained to believe that our medical system is the best, often more traditional cultures consider American medicine valuable only for treating the symptoms of disease, while believing traditional medicine is needed to cure it. To offer appropriate and effective care to today's diverse patient population, it is important not only to know the best that Western medicine has to offer, but also to consider what culturally rooted, traditional beliefs a patient may have about the causes and cures of illness.

Introduction

This guide is designed to assist healthcare professionals and staff in understanding the needs, expectations, and behaviors of multicultural patient populations. The information contained in the guide has been limited to "need to know" essential information and organized in an easily accessible format so that caregivers can consult it "on the spot." Although intended for direct caregivers, the guide will also prove helpful to office personnel, particularly those responsible for setting appointments or having the initial contact with patients. Additional sources are listed for those who wish to learn more about a particular cultural group.

This guide contains general tips on communicating with persons from other cultures and specific information to improve the caregiver's ability to interact successfully with patients from specific ethnic and/or cultural groups. Also included are guidelines for using interpreters, for communicating with limited-English-speaking patients, and for integrating the patients' cultural beliefs and traditional health practices with the caregiver's treatment plan in order to encourage compliance. The guide provides a useful tool for all medical personnel and institutions to understand culturally diverse populations and provide culturally appropriate, high-quality care.

Avoiding Stereotypes

Just as one cannot predict with certainty whether a particular member of a family with a history of heart disease will suffer from that disease, one cannot assume that an individual from a specific racial or cultural background will necessarily reflect the customs, traditions, and beliefs often associated with that race or culture. Many other factors, such as place of birth, family history, and social, economic, and educational status, affect the degree to which any individual will subscribe to the health beliefs and practices described in this guide.

Urban versus rural upbringing, length of time in the United States, level of acculturation to the life and ways of mainstream American culture—these are just a few of the many other cultural, social, and individual factors that will affect the extent to which specific cultural beliefs and practices shape a patient's approach to medical care.

It is, nevertheless, essential that the caregiver ascertain the extent to which a patient subscribes to traditional and/or modern health beliefs and practices in order to correctly assess his or her presenting symptoms and provide an appropriate treatment plan.

Tips for Avoiding Treating Patients as Stereotypes

Tip 1. **Find out where the patient is on the continuum of health beliefs and practices often associated with his or her population group.** It is a mistake to assume that because someone belongs to a particular ethnic, racial, or cultural group, they will necessarily believe or follow any or all of the practices described in this book or generally attributed to his or her primary group. By asking the following questions, caregivers will be better able to determine the degree of influence membership in a particular ethnic, racial, and/or cultural group has on the individual patient's health/illness beliefs and practices. This information will help the caregiver determine how to adjust treatment plans to appropriately meet that patient's needs and expectations.*

Personal Background

1. Where were you born?
2. If you were born in the United States, where were your parents born?
3. If you were born outside the United States, how old were you when you came to this country?
4. What were the circumstances surrounding your move from the country of your birth to the United States? Were the circumstances happy or sad? Why?
5. Did either you or members of your family come here because of war, famine, or other difficult or frightening situations that existed in your own country?
6. What were your most difficult experiences during your move to this country and your first days here?
7. What is the last grade of school that you completed? Was your schooling in the United States or abroad?
8. When you were ill as a child, who took care of you?
9. If you had a stuffy nose, a cough, or the flu, what did that person do to help you get better? Who did your relative(s) call if the illness persisted or was serious?
10. How long have you lived in this area?
11. Are there many [insert people from patient's group, such as Latinos, Chinese, Serbs] living in your present neighborhood?

Personal Data

1. What's going on in your life now?
2. What kinds of social, community, and/or religious activities do you regularly participate in?
3. Do members of your community help out when you or others become ill?
4. When you are ill, who takes care of you?
5. What does that person do to help you get better?

Consultation and Treatment

1. Why have you come in to see us today?
2. What do you think has caused this condition?
3. How long have you had it?
4. Before coming here, have you tried any measures to improve this condition? What have you tried?
5. Have you consulted anyone else, such as a relative, pharmacist, herbalist, spiritual leader, or other physicians or nurses, about this condition?
6. What did that person advise?
7. Did you take their advice? How successful do you think it was?
8. Do you plan to continue seeing that person or using that method along with what I suggest?
9. Are you eating, drinking, or otherwise taking anything to help you at this time?
10. What do you hope I will be able to do for you today?
11. How are decisions regarding health or healthcare made in your family? Would you like me to discuss my findings or my recommendations for treatment with anyone other than you?

*The development of this series of questions was influenced by the article by A. Kleinman, L. Eisenberg, and B. Good, "Culture, Illness, and Care: Clinical Lessons from Anthropologic and Cross-Cultural Research," *Annals of Internal Medicine* 88, no. 2 (February 1978): 251–8.

12. How much do you want to know about the results of my examination or any related tests? Should I find anything seriously wrong, would you want to know about it? Would you prefer to know only about my suggestions for making you feel better, such as a treatment plan?

13. Are there any particular family, financial, or other conditions that might make it difficult for you to return for further treatment or follow a recommended plan of medication or treatment?*

Tip 2. **Refrain from "judging" any of the beliefs or practices the patient reveals during the interview above.** In order to establish a trusting relationship between caregiver and patient, it is essential to acknowledge the patient's beliefs without criticism. Should the patient indicate that he or she engages in an unbeneficial but harmless practice, do not advise that the practice be abandoned. Should the patient disclose using an intervention or practice that is contraindicative, explain that it should be discontinued because it would be too strong if taken/done along with your recommended medication or treatment plan.

Tip 3. **Honor the patient's decision-making processes.** If the patient's replies to the questions above indicate that others such as family, religious leaders, or traditional healers are involved in his or her healthcare decisions, it is strongly recommended that these persons be included or acknowledged in any decisions that the patient is being asked to make. Although the American model of healthcare is based upon the autonomy of patient decisions, this may not be appropriate for patients who view decision making as a collective endeavor.

Tip 4. **Negotiate, don't dictate, your treatment plan.** Often patients, who view the caregiver or caregiving institution with great deference and authority, may appear to agree with a treatment plan that they in fact cannot or do not intend to follow. This is because they feel that it is more "polite" not to argue with authority. Therefore, before prescribing a treatment plan that requires following a particular daily diet plan or change of activities, find out what the patient usually eats or does—then make suggestions for changes one at a time, without overly criticizing the patient's present habits and always asking the patient if or how these changes can be made. It is also a good idea to ask the patient what or who might interfere with making any of these changes.

Tip 5. **Modify both your personal and your medical approach according to where the patient is on the continuum of health beliefs and practices.** The results of the interview suggested above may indicate that the patient is more comfortable within the framework of the American approach to treatment or, more likely, that he or she is influenced by a combination of traditional and modern healthcare beliefs and practices.

*Other questionnaires can be found in Rachel E. Spector, *Cultural Diversity in Health and Illness*, 6th ed. (Upper Saddle River, N.J.: Pearson Prentice Hall, 2004), and the article by L.S. Lieberman, et al., "Women's Health Care: Cross-Cultural Encounters within the Medical System," *Journal of the Florida Medical Association* 84, no.6 (August/September 1997): 364–73.

A Guide, Not a Rulebook

The cultural and health information presented is intended as a guide, not a rulebook. No strict profile of a particular patient's beliefs, practices, or communication styles should be drawn solely on the basis of this information, nor should the information be used as a recipe for the treatment of individual patients of any cultural group.

What this guide provides is an extra dimension in the caregiver's body of knowledge. This information should be drawn upon judiciously in considering possible diagnoses and treatments, investigating responses to medications or treatments, and evaluating patients' behavior.

The population groups discussed in this section are broadly labeled African Americans, American Indians and Alaska Natives, Asians, Hispanics/Latinos, Middle Easterners, and emigrés from the former Soviet bloc countries. In some ways, these terms conceal more than they reveal. As the reader will see, each group comprises many different cultures, nationalities, histories, and heritages. Statistically, these labels and categories are useful organizers of beliefs and traits with more similarities than differences; however, the caregiver must remember that statistics do not apply to individuals.

CULTURAL OVERVIEW

African Americans

African Americans are the second largest minority group in the United States, comprising about 12.3 percent of the total U.S. population according to the 2000 U.S. Census, a figure projected to rise to almost 14.6 percent by the year 2050.* African Americans have almost as long a history in the United States as the earliest White settlers, and a longer history than many immigrant groups. Because of this lengthy American heritage, it is easy for both African Americans and White Americans to assume that only one factor—skin color—distinguishes them from one another.

In the healthcare environment, this assumption can have serious consequences. The belief that to ensure appropriate care all the caregiver has to do is ignore skin color and proceed to the usual treatments can sometimes lead to failure, anger, and frustration on the part of both patient and caregiver. This approach ignores the fact that cultural differences may exist and can result in vastly different expectations regarding the nature of quality care and the elements of a pleasant, nurturing caregiver/patient relationship.

In fact, many African Americans reflect cultural roots that include elements of African healing, medicine of the Civil War South, European medical and anatomical folklore, West Indies voodoo religion, fundamentalist Christianity, and other belief systems. While a great deal of the information presented here may be unfamiliar to many African American physicians and patients, these beliefs and practices may directly or indirectly influence the healthcare behavior of some of the African Americans under the caregiver's treatment.

African American communities have become very diverse, especially with the recent arrival of people from Haiti, the Caribbean, and Africa. While this discussion is limited to an overview of beliefs and practices of U.S.-born African Americans, it is important to note that some of the beliefs and practices of these

* Census 2000 data on race are not directly comparable with data from the 1990 census or earlier censuses because in 2000, for the first time, respondents could report one or more races. The data in this section reflect the more conservative figures representing respondents who reported only one race. The figures for Hispanics/Latinos are not affected by this change, as they are based on ethnicity rather than race.

African Americans have been influenced by beliefs that have arrived with recent immigrants. Furthermore, because diverse African American groups frequently interact, many African American immigrants are also influenced by the beliefs described herein.

American Indians and Alaska Natives

The term *American Indian* refers to members of Indian tribal nations who live in the United States. The term *Alaska Native* refers to the Eskimo and Aleut populations. *Native American*, a term that has become unpopular among American Indian groups, refers to American Indians, Eskimos, and Aleuts as one racial and ethnic group.

If Eskimo and Aleut populations are included, Native Americans numbered 2.47 million in 2000, or 0.9 percent of the U.S. population, and their numbers are growing rapidly. The Native American group as a whole is expected to reach 5 million by 2065, comprising 1.1 percent of the population, a fact reflecting both the greater efficiency of the Census Bureau in counting Indians living on reservations and trust lands, and the comparative youth and fertility of the Native American population. In 2000, the median age of Native Americans was 28, with 33.9 percent under 18. This group is extremely diverse, with more than 500 (300 American Indian alone) distinct Indian nations and Alaska Native villages, each with its own unique language, tribal laws, and culture.

Of the American Indian population, most live west of the Mississippi River, with the majority living in Oklahoma, California, Arizona, and New Mexico. The poverty rate is higher than the national average. In 2003, 23.2 percent of the American Indian population lived below the poverty line, unchanged from the previous year, compared to the national average of 12.5 percent.

Many American Indians continue to practice tribal religions and traditional medicine. One study reported that 70 percent of Navajo living on the reservation use traditional healers, while another found that approximately 28 percent of Indians living in Milwaukee and the San Francisco Bay area continued to use traditional practitioners.

Asians

In 2000, the Census Bureau reported that Asians made up 3.6 percent of the total U.S. population. Predictions are that this population group will more than double and comprise 8.0 percent of the U.S. population by 2050.

There are five major Asian population groups in the United States: Chinese (including people from Taiwan, Hong Kong, and mainland China), Filipino, Korean, Japanese, and Southeast Asian (including people from Laos, Cambodia, Vietnam, and Thailand). Although also inhabitants of the continent of Asia, people from India, Pakistan, Malaysia, and Indonesia are not included in this classification, since these groups are racially different from the five groups noted above.

Although Asian groups are very diverse in terms of culture, language, etiquette, and rules for interaction, a common thread of Confucian, Buddhist, and Taoist thought links their healthcare beliefs and practices.

The oldest and largest Asian population is Chinese. With a population of over 2,400,000 according to the 2000 U.S. Census, Chinese Americans make up almost 0.9 percent of the total population. The second largest group of Asians in the United States is Filipino Americans, with a population of 1,850,000, or almost 0.7 percent of the U.S. population. Next in order are the Southeast Asian Americans, Korean Americans, and Japanese Americans.

Hispanics/Latinos

The term *Hispanic* is an artificial designation that was created by the U.S. Census Bureau in 1970 as an ethnic category for persons who identify themselves as being of Spanish origin. Unlike other Census Bureau designations, *Hispanic* denotes neither race nor color, and a Hispanic may be White, Black, or American Indian. The term *Latino* first appeared in the U.S. Census in 2000, when all respondents were asked to identify whether or not they were of *Spanish/Hispanic/Latino* ethnicity.

The Hispanic/Latino population is now the largest and fastest growing minority in the United States. According to the 2000 U.S. Census, Hispanics/Latinos made up 12.5 percent of the population and are expected to comprise 24.5 percent of the total U.S. population by 2050.Hispanics may include (1) Mexican Americans/Chicanos, (2) Puerto Ricans/Boricuas, (3) Hispanos (U.S. Hispanics who identify themselves as "Spanish"), (4) Cuban Americans, and (5) Latinos (Hispanics from countries other than those already mentioned). Terms other than *Hispanic* may be preferred. For example, many Mexican Americans prefer *Chicano,* Puerto Ricans may prefer *Boricuas,* while others may prefer the more general term, *Latino.*

The classification *Hispanic/Latino* includes people of many different origins and cultures. Because the pattern of interactions among Spanish settlers, indigenous Indian populations, and African slaves differed across the many Latin American countries, the resulting diversity in these countries is considerable. Therefore, although there is a unifying thread of language and some cultural similarities inherited from the Spanish settlers, there is also tremendous variety within the Hispanic community. In the discussion of Hispanic health beliefs and practices, those that are common to all Hispanics are emphasized to guide health practitioners in providing appropriate care.

Middle Easterners

The diverse groups of people often referred to under the general term "Middle Easterner" include Arab Americans, Egyptian Americans, and Iranian Americans. It is hard to give the exact number of people from the Middle East living in the United States because these groups are counted as White by the Census Bureau. However, it is estimated that there are at least 3,500,000 Arab Americans, including half a million Egyptian Americans, and about 1,000,000 Iranian Americans living in the United States.

Arab Americans are those people who speak Arabic or are descendants of Arabic-speaking populations. While Egyptian Americans speak Arabic, both their language and culture are as different from other Arab groups as the British are from Americans. Armenians who have immigrated (or are descendants of immigrants) from Arabic-speaking countries have not been included in this discussion because most have maintained their ethnic and cultural ties with Armenia. Although Iranian Americans, speakers of Farsi (sometimes called Persian), are of Indo-European rather than Semitic origin, they have been included because of the strong cultural similarities with these other groups. Israelis, who also come from the geographic area referred to as the Middle East, have not been included in this discussion. Most Jewish Israelis living in the United States are of European origin and have healthcare beliefs that have little in common with those of the other groups discussed.

In spite of the fact that there are major similarities in culture and health beliefs and practices of patients who come from countries loosely referred to as the "Middle East," caregivers are advised to inquire about what country the patient comes from, what religion he or she follows, and what language is the primary language of the home. As religious factors may play an important part in health beliefs and practices, caregivers should take care not to assume that every Middle Eastern patient is a follower of Islam. The majority of Middle Easterners living in the United States are Muslim, but many are not. They may be of Christian, Coptic Christian, or Jewish faith. Language backgrounds are also diverse. Those who come from Algeria, Bahrain, Egypt, Iraq, Jordan, Morocco, Saudi Arabia, Syria, United Arab Emirates, or one of the other Arab countries are likely to understand Arabic, but they may speak Berber, Egyptian, Kurdish, or French as their primary language. Those from the non-Arab countries, on the other hand, may not know Arabic and speak Persian (Farsi), Azerbaijani, or Hebrew. Asking about the patient's country of origin and language is one of the first steps in building a successful caregiver/patient relationship.

Emigrés from the Former Soviet Bloc Countries

The population groups discussed under this category include emigrés from the former Soviet Union, former Yugoslavia (Bosnia), and Poland. These groups have little in common culturally and there is a great diversity in religions. Their religious backgrounds may be Jewish, Catholic, Protestant, Pentecostal Christian, Orthodox Christian, or Muslim. While older members may follow these religious traditions, many of those who grew up during the period when communist governments actively discouraged religion have no formal religious beliefs. Still, because of long histories of religious strife, members of these populations tend to group themselves on the basis of these religious backgrounds.

While some of the immigrants from Russia and Poland came in earlier waves of immigration, others are recent newcomers. In 2003, Russia and Poland ranked tenth and sixteenth, respectively, among the top twenty countries of origin for immigrants to the United States. Many Bosnian emigrés have arrived directly from Bosnia or from Germany or other countries in Europe over the past ten years. Bosnia-Herzegovina ranked eighth among the top twenty countries of origin for immigrants to the United States in 2002. Although there was an attempt to include the most recent emigrés from the former Yugoslavia, the Kosovars (mostly ethnic Albanians), no concrete information could be obtained about this newly arriving population.

In spite of the diversity of culture and religion, the communist economy created a commonality of attitudes regarding the balance between personal and governmental roles and responsibilities regarding healthcare. Under the communist system, healthcare, regardless of the quality of care, was considered the right of every citizen. In addition, the health systems in Russia, Yugoslavia, and Poland were similar enough to have generated common expectations and approaches to dealing with illness and the need for medical treatment.

Chapter 1

Tips for Successful Caregiver/ Patient Interaction across Cultures

The following sets of tips relating to language and culture will help maximize communication and build trust between you and your patient. These tips won't solve every communication difficulty, but they will increase the patient's sense of trust, and lower the frustration that both you and your patient feel when a "cultural or linguistic wall" seems to separate you!

Tips for Improving the Cross-Cultural Caregiver/Patient Relationship

Tip 1. **Don't treat the patient in the same manner you would want to be treated.** The Golden Rule of "Do unto others..." does not work across cultures! Culture determines the rules for polite, caring behavior and will thus formulate the patient's concept of a satisfactory caregiver/patient relationship.

Tip 2. **Begin by being more formal with patients who were born in another culture.** The use of first names as a means of "putting someone at ease," demonstrating respect and a sense of equality, is unique to the United States. In most countries, a greater distance between caregiver and patient is maintained throughout the relationship. Except when treating children or very young adults, it's best to use the patient's last name when addressing them. The caregiver must determine the correct form of address. Is the name the patient gives first likely to be his or her first name or family name? When in doubt, both nurses and physicians should introduce themselves by their surnames and ask, "By which name would you like me to call you?" or "What name would you like me to use when I speak to you?"

Tip 3. **Don't be "put off" if the patient fails to "look you in the eye" or ask questions about the treatment.** Both may be due to the patient's culturally prescribed way of showing respect for your knowledge and position. A patient who refuses to look you in the eye may be doing so, not to hide information, but to show his or her respect. In many cultures it is considered disrespectful to look directly at another person (especially one in authority) or to make them "lose face" by asking questions. One of the reasons that Americans are so quick to address one another by first names is because in our culture it demonstrates equality and lack of social and/or occupational ranks. These values are not shared by everyone. In many cultures, caregivers, especially physicians, are considered authority figures who have high social and educational status. These "distances" are greatly valued. Should a caregiver treat a patient as an equal, the caregiver would lose status in the patient's eyes. The caregiver would also lose status in the patient's eyes by attempting to include the patient in the medical decision-making process. Patients of many cultures have been taught to place the physician (and, often, the nurse) on a pedestal. They are considered the "knowers" to whom common people look for decisions regarding matters of health. Patients may expect the physician to tell them firmly what must be done. Should the caregiver consult with the patient or try to share responsibility for decisions regarding care, the patient may fear that the caregiver neither knows enough nor has enough experience to solve his or her health problems.

Tip 4. **Don't make *any* assumptions regarding the patient's concepts about the ways to maintain health, the causes of illness, or the means to prevent or cure illness.** Adopt a line of questioning that will help you determine some of the patient's central beliefs about health, illness, and illness prevention.

Tip 5. **Allow the patient to be open and honest with you by not discounting or laughing at beliefs that are not held by our Western biomedical tradition.** Often patients are afraid to tell Western caregivers that they are visiting a faith or folk healer, or are taking an alternative medicine concurrently with Western treatment because in the past they have experienced ridicule by doing so.

Tip 6. **Don't discount the possible effect of the belief in the supernatural on the patient's health and wellbeing.** If the patient believes that the illness has been caused by *embrujado* (bewitchment) or someone casting an evil eye on him or her, or as a punishment for something that has been done, that patient is not likely to take any responsibility for his or her cure. This may result in the patient's failure to either follow medical advice or comply with the treatment plan.

Tip 7. **Make your questioning indirect concerning the patient's belief in the supernatural or use of nontraditional forms of cure** by saying something like, "Many of my patients from [name of country] believe [*or* do *or* visit]... Do you?"

Tip 8. **Try to ascertain the value of involving the entire family in the treatment.** In many cultures, medical decisions are made by the immediate family or even the extended family. If you can involve the family in both the decision-making process and the treatment plan, there is a greater likelihood of gaining the patient's compliance with the course of treatment.

Tip 9. **Be cautious around issues of "informed consent."** Informed consent, which most Americans have come to take for granted, is an almost uniquely American concept. Sometimes, when dealing with patients from other cultures, giving them a full description of negative possibilities yet asking them to sign a consent form may be viewed as demonstrating a lack of caring and even as cruelty. In Navajo culture, for example, where the word is thought to precipitate the deed and not the other way around, even a discussion of possible negative outcomes may be considered a form of "making the bad happen." In many cultures and countries, a patient would never be told a negative prognosis. Instead, a family member (possibly an elder) would be told, and the patient would be given only minimal information. When one Polish-born and trained physician was still living in Poland, he watched an American movie in which an American physician informed his patient that she had inoperable uterine cancer. He was sure that it simply reflected Hollywood's lack of knowledge about the medical profession because "no physician would ever tell his patient she was going to die." After immigrating to the States, this same physician soon learned that the movie he had seen gave an accurate account of our standard medical practice.

Tip 10. **Be very restrained in relating bad news or in explaining in detail the many complications that may result from a particular course of treatment.** The "need to know" is a uniquely American trait. In many other cultures, placing oneself in the doctor's hands represents an act of trust and a desire to transfer the responsibility for the choice of treatment upon the physician. Therefore, it is advisable to watch for and respect signs that the patient has learned as much as he or she is able to deal with.

Tip 11. **Whenever possible, try to incorporate into your treatment plan the elements of the patient's folk medication and folk beliefs that are not specifically contraindicated.** This will encourage the patient's development of trust in your treatment and help ensure that your treatment plan is followed.

Tips for Determining the Individual Etiquette, Beliefs, and Practices of Patients from Other Cultures

Tip 1. **Introduce yourself formally, using title and last name, and ask the patient how he or she wishes to be addressed.** Some patients will expect anyone who is not a close member of their family to call them by their family name.

Tip 2. **Ask the patient what he or she believes has caused the illness.** Do not mock the patient or laugh if the patient believes his or her illness was caused by a curse, an evil eye, or a spirit. Ask them to explain to you how or why they think this happened.

Tip 3. **Ask the patient how they think the illness or complaint can best be cured.** What would they do about this illness if they were back in their home culture? If the patient believes the complaint has supernatural causes, he or she will probably believe that only a supernatural cure will work. Encourage the patient to follow any of his or her culture's traditional procedures as long as they will not harm the patient or be contraindicated by the medication you plan to prescribe.

Tip 4. **Ask the patient if he or she has consulted anyone else about the complaint prior to coming to you.** Try to learn whether or not the patient has consulted a community elder, a healer, a fortune teller, or an herbalist. If the answer is "yes," try to find out what herbs, teas, or cures have been advised and whether or not the patient thinks they are working. It is very important not to ridicule these treatments or to try to convince the patient that they won't work!

Tip 5. **Ask the patient how medical decisions are made in his or her culture** and whether he or she wishes to consult with a relative or member of the community prior to making a decision. If the patient wishes to discuss the decision with someone else, it is best to do so prior to your explanation of possible treatment plans and procedures.

Tip 6. **Never assume that a patient will be familiar with a particular type of medical test or procedure.** Even a woman who has had several children may not have had a vaginal exam and a man may never have been asked about his sexual behavior. Some patients may not have ever been asked to disrobe for an examination.

Tip 7. **Before prescribing a dietary regime, ask the patient what he or she usually eats, as well as how often and what time meals are eaten.** Try to find out whether the patient subscribes to the "hot"/"cold" theory of disease and, if so, whether the complaint is considered "hot" or "cold." A "hot" medication or food should never be advised for a "hot" complaint nor a "cold" medication or food for a "cold" one. It is also important to learn about beliefs in lucky or unlucky numbers. If a patient believes four is an unlucky number, try not to prescribe medication to be taken four times a day.

Tip 8. **Be prepared to accept the fact that excellence in care will mean very different things to patients of different cultures.** Don't try to treat the patient as you would want to be treated. Try to ascertain how he or she wants to be treated and make every effort to treat that patient accordingly.

Tips for Communicating Directly with Limited-English-Speaking Patients

Tip 1. **Speak slowly, not loudly.** Remember that the patient is hard of *understanding*, not hearing! A loud voice implies anger, and in most cultures the physician/caregiver holds a very high position of respect and authority. When patients feel that the caregiver is angry, they tend to become nervous and answer questions in the way that they think will please the caregiver and dispel his or her anger, rather than give the true picture of their complaint.

Tip 2. **Face the patient and make extensive use of gestures, pictures, and facial expressions.** By the same token, watch the patient's face, eyes, and body language carefully. When these don't agree with the patient's words, or the patient's eyes or facial expression doesn't clearly indicate that what has been said is understood—double-check carefully!

Tip 3. **Avoid difficult and uncommon words and idiomatic expressions.** American English is fraught with idioms such as "right on target," "in the nick of time," "kill two birds with one stone," and so forth. Americans also use idioms to demonstrate friendliness, respect, or equality. While most idioms are perfectly simple and comprehensible even to the youngest American-born patient, they tend to confuse, intimidate, and alienate most immigrants.

Tip 4. **Don't "muddy the waters" with unnecessary words or information!** More is not better! Keep what you say simple. Strip the information you give down to bare essentials. Remember, too: Not all patients expect or want all the facts about their illness explained in full or want you to tell them the truth about the prognosis for recovery. In most other cultures a poor prognosis is hidden not only from the patient, but often from the family, too.

Tip 5. **Organize what you say for easy access.** Use short, simple sentences, starting with the subject, followed, as closely as possible, by the verb and a simple object. A good rule of thumb is that people tend to remember information in an inverted bell curve—what is said at the beginning and end is remembered best, while the information in the middle is missed or quickly forgotten. Put your information where it counts!

Tip 6. **Rephrase and summarize often.** Try to say the same thing or ask the same question in at least two or three different ways.

Tip 7. **Don't ask questions that can be answered by "yes" or "no."** The patient's answer will only tell you whether or not the question has been heard—not whether it has been understood. If you phrase questions in a way that requires the patient to respond with information (i.e., by beginning them with *what, where, when, why,* or *how*), they can only reply sensibly if they have understood the question.

Tip 8. **Check *your* understanding of the patient by paraphrasing what he or she has said.** Remember: Questions like "Did you say...?" will not get accurate results—try to ask a question that requires information rather than just a "yes" or "no"!

Tip 9. **Check the *concept* behind the word!** The patient may interpret even the simplest instructions, such as "Keep the baby warm," "Wash the wound regularly," or "Eat a balanced diet," in a radically different way than you intended. Words only function as a means of calling up ideas and concepts gained through prior experience. When dealing with people who come from a different culture and lifestyle, it's important to remember that, although a person may have learned the English word for something, they are probably associating it with experiences more closely tied to their cultural experience than to ours.

Tip 10. **Don't burden the patient with decisions he or she is not prepared to make.** Unlike most American patients, who wish to be given *all* the options so that they can make an informed choice for themselves, people from most other cultures tend to believe in the "mystique" of the physician and the "healer's art." The physician is expected to review the case and *tell* them what to do. *Asking* the patient often destroys the patient's faith in the knowledge and expertise of the physician and the medical institution!

Tips for Improving the Effectiveness of Interpreters

Tip 1. **Brief the interpreter** first by summarizing what you will say to the patient and emphasizing the key information you wish to impart.

Tip 2. **Explain information/ask questions in two or three different ways.** Don't be afraid of repeating yourself. Try to choose different words and expressions with each explanation or question. This will help rule out misunderstanding.

Tip 3. **Avoid long or complicated sentences.** Be concise and try to avoid superfluous words or ideas.

Tip 4. **Keep it short!** Don't talk for more than one or two minutes without stopping to allow the interpreter to explain what you have said to the patient.

Tip 5. **Allow the interpreter "thought time."** The professionally trained interpreter will try to capture the essence of what you mean rather than simply translate word-for-word. Sometimes it takes a bit of time to convey the same meaning in a language with an entirely different structure and communication pattern.

Tip 6. **Don't interrupt!** Interrupting the interpreter while he/she is talking to the patient may cause him/her to "lose face" in the patient's eyes, to lose the train of thought, or even to forget some vital information.

Tip 7. **Don't be impatient!** Permit the interpreter to use as much time as is necessary to clarify a point.

Tip 8. **Allow for the "directness of English."** Don't be concerned if the interpreter takes five to ten minutes to "summarize" what you have said in two minutes. Don't be concerned if the patient talks for five to ten minutes and the interpreter tells you what has been said in two minutes!

Tip 9. **Utilize/read gestures and facial expressions.** Arrange yourself so that you, the patient, and the interpreter are visible to one another. Use lots of gestures and facial expressions when you speak *through* the interpreter. Watch the patient's eyes and facial expression—both when you speak and when the interpreter speaks. Look for signs of comprehension, confusion, agreement, or disagreement.

Tip 10. **Remember that "culture" may cause even a professional interpreter to modify what you or the patient has said.** Clarify with the interpreter whether it's OK to discuss sexual or other "delicate issues," give bad news to the patient, and so forth. Ask the interpreter the best way to broach these subjects with the patient or family.

Tips for Improving Patient Satisfaction and Compliance by Integrating Cultural or Folk Medical Practices and Beliefs into Your Treatment Plan

Tip 1. **Learn about your patients' basic health/illness beliefs and practices by asking patients directly or indirectly about:**

Food and Diet
- What constitutes their basic diet?
- What are their food preferences?
- Do they believe that certain foods/beverages are healthy or unhealthy? Question your patient carefully about food beliefs at "special times" such as before/after surgery, during menstruation or childbirth.

Medication
- Do they take herbs or tonics? If so, what are they? Who recommended them?
- Are certain forms of medication (e.g., pills, suppositories, liquids) preferred over others?
- Who is responsible for healthcare decision making?

Other Forms of Care
- Have they ever visited a healer, a "doctor" of folk or traditional medicine, or an herbalist?
- Have any of their friends or family ever visited one?

The Body
- How do they view the roles of the specific bodily organs or parts you wish to treat?
- Do they believe that there is a direct relationship between emotions and disease (e.g., *fright* in Chinese culture, *susto* in Hispanic culture)?
- Does their culture have any religious or folk prohibitions to surgery, blood loss, or blood transfusions?

Superstition
- Do they, or others of their religion or culture, hold any special beliefs about lucky or unlucky numbers or signs or days?
- Are there any beliefs or taboos against the caregiver touching the top of the head or any other parts of the patient's body?
- Do they believe that supernatural powers can cause illness?

Tip 2. **Consider which of the above beliefs would not interfere with your plan of treatment or be contraindicated.** Try to integrate as many of your patient's beliefs as possible into your plan. If the belief or activity isn't contraindicated, allowing your patient to utilize it will build a strong bond of trust, confidence, and patient satisfaction.

Tip 3. **Avoid, whenever possible, a treatment plan that conflicts with the patient's beliefs and lifestyle.**
Consider the following questions:

- Is your standard blood test really necessary?
- Does the patient need to drink fruit juices that might be classified as "cold"? What foods or drinks in the patient's regular diet could be substituted?
- Does the patient need to eat "slippery foods," which the Chinese believe might make the baby "fall out" prematurely, during pregnancy?
- Can "slush" be made from a combination of prescribed foods and medications?
- Does that Asian patient have to take pills four times a day or be placed on the fourth floor of the hospital?
- Is there any real medical reason to forbid the relatives from bringing the patient's favorite foods?
- Can you postpone doing a Pap smear on a Hispanic patient because she is menstruating?
- Can medication be regulated by connecting time of dosage to an activity rather than to a specific hour in cultures that have very loose concepts about time?

Tips for Diet and Nutrition Assessment and Counseling

Tip 1. **Learn something about the traditional diet and lifestyle of the cultures to which some of your patients belong.** Remember that not all of the patients from that culture conform to that traditional picture, but it will give you a reference point for asking questions to ascertain the individual patient's eating habits. You might want to start a file or reference notebook of the traditional diets of cultural groups in your service area.

Tip 2. **Don't make any assumptions based on standard U.S. eating habits.** Even concepts such as what constitutes a meal versus a snack may vary greatly from culture to culture. Instead of asking the patient/client what he or she had for breakfast, ask more general questions such as, "What is the first thing you usually eat or drink when you get up in the morning? What time do you usually have it? What is the next time you usually have something to eat or drink? What kinds of things do you have?"

Tip 3. **Identify the specific dietary changes undergone by immigrants since coming to the United States.** For example, you might ask what the midday meal usually consisted of in the person's home country and what it consists of now. Ask which type of food the patient prefers, which type he or she believes to be more healthful, and why.

Tip 4. **Try to identify taboos about particular foods.** Ask whether there are any foods or drinks forbidden by the patient's religion or any foods he or she believes are "unclean" or "bad." Work with the patient to develop a dietary plan that is culturally appropriate and acceptable.

Tip 5. **Ask the person about beliefs in the special properties of certain foods.** Do some foods make one strong, make one smart, give good eyesight, give sexual strength? Do some cure or prevent certain illnesses? These questions may reveal some rather surprising belief systems! In December 1999, the *Chicago Tribune* reported a traffic in rats because some Mexican Americans believed in the healing power of eating field rats. Rats were reputed to be a great source of energy—especially for the weak and sick! It's best to make suggestions for viable substitutes rather than criticize these beliefs.

Tip 6. **When advising a patient that a change in dietary habits is necessary, try to negotiate changes that are healthful and appropriate** to the patient's cultural environment and lifestyle as well as individual likes and dislikes. Utilize patient education materials such as traditional food pyramids. Remember that traditional foods such as beans are often abandoned by ethnic groups because they are associated with poverty. Meat, on the other hand, may represent to them the affluence of America.

Tip 7. **Beware of the strong "pull" of a belief in fatalism in the unwillingness of some culturally diverse patients to change their diet and lifestyle.** Many culturally diverse patients believe that food choice or amount consumed has nothing to do with obesity or with diseases such as diabetes, high blood pressure, or high cholesterol. These diseases are often attributed to luck, God's will, or fate. A person's ability to control his or her health through lifestyle choices is a particularly Western concept. Convincing those who do not believe that the changes you suggest actually can and will improve their health requires your patience and understanding.

Tip 8. **There are biochemical reasons for some food choices or omissions in traditional diets.** One example is the absence of milk and milk products from the traditional Asian diet. This may be explained by the fact that as many as 75 percent of Asians and those of Asian descent are lactose intolerant. Alternative calcium sources are soybean curd, soy milk fortified with calcium, and seaweed in the Japanese diet.

DEVELOPING CULTURAL PERSPECTIVE

1. Refer to "Tips for Improving Patient Satisfaction and Compliance" on pages 6-7. Read and answer each of the questions about "Food and Diet," "The Body," and "Belief System" according to what you know about your own culture.

2. Refer to "Tips for Improving Patient Satisfaction and Compliance" on pages 6-7. Select any cultural group described in this book and read and answer each of the questions about "Food and Diet," "The Body," and "Belief System" appropriately for that group.

3. Compare your answers to #1 and #2 above. Are there similarities? Any differences?

4. Without referring back to the chapter, create a list of general communication guidelines that you can use to communicate with limited English-speaking patients. Compare your list to the text. Are there similarities? Any differences?

BLENDING PERSPECTIVES

1. Make a list of communication methods and facial expressions that are common across cultures. How many of these examples do you use effectively? How can you use these common factors to help make a foreign-born patient more comfortable?

2. Does the phrase "common courtesy" extend across cultures? How might your style of common courtesy help you with foreign-born patients? Could it hinder you? How?

Chapter 2

Providing Culture-Sensitive Healthcare to African Americans

Keys to a Good Professional Relationship with African American Patients

1. *Don't assume.* Although the classification "African American" refers to race or skin color, it also may involve noticeable cultural characteristics. Many African Americans grew up in a culture that is essentially a different America, and the English they speak amongst themselves is different from that spoken by White Americans. It is important to keep in mind that although many African Americans share similar childhood backgrounds and current lifestyles with White American caregivers, many may come from or live in neighborhoods so different from a White caregiver's experience that the lifestyle, communication patterns, and rules of acceptable behavior can be likened to those of persons from another country. Regardless of socioeconomic or educational status, being African American in this country involves cultural norms very different from those of the non-Hispanic Caucasian population. Although the majority of African Americans have, as a matter of survival, learned to "code switch" in many instances to get along in a primarily White environment, many have not. Furthermore, illness, pain, and fear for well-being may make the patient or patient's family forget to switch codes and operate within the confines of the dominant White culture. In most cases, the patient will feel more comfortable, more valued, and more satisfied with care when caregivers make the effort to adapt to the patient's needs and expectations rather than expect the patient to be willing and able to adapt to mainstream culture. Regardless of the race of the caregiver, no assumption should be made about the similarity or difference in background between the caregiver and the patient. With respect to health-related beliefs and practices, an African American patient may be as different from an African American caregiver as from a White, Latino, or Asian physician. On the other hand, an African American patient may be quite similar to the caregiver, regardless of the caregiver's race. It is the task of the caregiver to refrain from making assumptions based upon race, and to probe and listen carefully to the patient to determine the patient's healthcare expectations, beliefs, and practices.

2. *Ask for causes.* When taking the initial history and performing a physical examination, ask patients not only about their symptoms, but also if they believe they know what has caused the illness. Patients' answers may give caregivers information regarding whether they subscribe to a folk or magical belief system and what the basis of this folk or magical belief is.
3. *Listen without judgment.* It is essential during all stages of a consultation that the caregiver listen carefully and sympathetically. Refrain from expressing anything that might be interpreted as judgmental, patronizing, or ridiculing.

Health Problems and Concerns Common to Members of African American Communities

Some African Americans may have a tendency toward certain health concerns because of cultural (including lifestyle and dietary habits), economic, or genetic factors. Life expectancy for African Americans is 67.4 years, as compared to 75 years for Whites. Specific concerns include the following:

1. *Hypertension* morbidity and mortality rates are three to five times higher than for Whites.
2. *Diabetes* is 33 percent more prevalent than in Whites.
3. *Coronary heart disease* is more prevalent with African Americans than it is with Whites.
4. *Cancer,* despite an improvement in the mortality rate, remains a major health problem.
5. *AIDS* affects about three times as many African Americans as non–African Americans.
6. *Infant mortality* among African Americans is high, with low birth weight and SIDS accounting for a large percentage of deaths.
7. *Sickle cell anemia* is a genetic disorder found almost exclusively in African Americans. Only 50 percent of children born with sickle cell anemia live to adulthood; others die before age 20, and many who do live suffer chronic and irreversible complications. Parents who are both AS heterozygotes should be informed that there is a 25 percent chance that their children will be born with sickle cell anemia. The disease can be diagnosed during the first trimester of pregnancy by DNA analysis. If the fetus is an SS homozygote, parents and caregivers may wish to discuss the viability of the pregnancy. Because the disorder is so debilitating to children, women who carry the gene for the disease may wish to consider a wide range of contraceptive options, including sterilization; the caregiver should be prepared for such discussions.
8. *Lactose intolerance* is common in African Americans (as well as in Asians, Africans, and Mexican Americans).

Physiologic Assessment of African Americans

1. Skin assessment is best done in indirect sunlight.
2. Pallor may be identified by an absence of underlying red tones. Brown skin tends to appear yellow-brown and black skin tends to appear ashen.
3. Erythema can be detected only by palpitation. The skin is warm, tight, and edematous in the inflamed area. Deeper tissues are hard.
4. Cyanosis may best be observed in facial skin, the earlobes, the nail beds, and around the mouth. Pressure applied to the nail beds or earlobes can be used to determine normal or slow return of color.
5. Jaundice can be seen in a generalized yellowing of the sclera. Because the normal yellow pigmentation found in dark-skinned individuals tends to be concentrated in the inner and outer canthi of the eyes and in the stool, blood tests may be needed to confirm the presence of jaundice.

Demographics and Health Profile of African Americans

The results of the 2000 U.S. Census show that African Americans comprise 12.3 percent of the total population. African American life expectancy at birth is 6 years shorter than that of Whites (70 years vs. 76 years) and 2 years shorter at age 65. According to the Commonwealth Fund Health Care Quality Survey (see "Sources for Further Reading"), access to health care is severely affected by higher poverty rates and high health insurance rates (about one in three African Americans aged 18–64 is uninsured). More African Americans than Whites live with chronic diseases and, according to this report, African Americans are more likely to have had negative healthcare experiences. Many feel that they would have received better care if they were of a different race or ethnicity.

Folk Beliefs of Some African Americans about Health and Illness That Can Affect Care and Treatment

Good health, although considered a matter of good fortune, results when one takes good care of oneself and makes sure that the body, mind, and soul remain in harmony with nature. Illness occurs when this balance is disturbed and is cured when harmony is restored. Because of the conviction that any illness can be cured if only the correct cause and appropriate cure are found, patients may not accept any diagnosis of a terminal disease or a chronic illness, but may instead continue to search for a different doctor, a new medicine, another treatment—including, perhaps, a folk or faith healer.

Patients who are told that they must take a particular medicine for life (e.g., for hypertension or diabetes) may be noncompliant because they are afraid that the true cause of the illness has not been found and the medicine is only a cover-up for the physician's not knowing how to cure them. They may also fear that too much medication for one illness may tip the balance in the opposite direction (for example, a patient taking medicine for high blood pressure too long may begin to suffer from low blood pressure).

The beliefs described below are prevalent in some, but not all, African American populations. While these beliefs may be unfamiliar to many African American physicians and patients, they may influence the healthcare behavior of a substantial number of patients (including those who are totally unaware of the origin of a particular belief). For this reason, the caregiver should be familiar with them. According to Snow (1974), the elements of African American folk medicine form "a coherent medical system and not a ragtag collection of isolated superstitions." To those who follow these beliefs, the system "makes just as much sense... as the principles of orthodox medicine do to the graduate of an accredited medical school."

1. *Belief in the forces of nature.* There is a direct connection between the human body and the forces of nature. Thus, dates, zodiacal signs, and numbers affect everyday behaviors and activities and should be taken into account in making decisions about health care and many other aspects of life.
2. *Use of sources such as* The Farmer's Almanac *for making healthcare decisions.* The Farmer's Almanac is used by many African Americans and Whites in the South as a guide for interpreting the effects of the phases of the moon, the position of the planets, and the seasons of the year on natural phenomena. If the *Almanac* is a reliable guide to planting, harvesting, and animal care, it is equally useful in determining the best dates to have a tooth filled (during the moon's decrease) or pulled (during its increase); the time to wean a baby; and the amount of self-medication to take for a particular illness, and when to take it. Patients who use the *Almanac* or other sources that explain zodiacal signs

to manage their health will probably not disclose this information to caregivers, either for fear of being ridiculed or because this belief is totally separated in the mind of the patient from biomedicine. Caregivers must listen carefully for comments that might indicate such beliefs and then ask the patient or the patient's family indirectly about them.

3. *Numbers that are thought to be either lucky or unlucky.* The numbers three and nine are thought to be especially powerful, and they are used frequently in deciding on the dosage for home remedies (e.g., taking three tablespoonsful three times a day for nine days) and magical rituals (e.g., identifying nine signs, saying a chant nine times, praying for nine days). While these rituals and remedies are being performed, the person is considered especially vulnerable to illnesses caused by "cold" (see below), and may avoid bathing because water conducts cold into the body.

4. *Humoral theory,* based on Aristotelian and early European medical beliefs, is a part of the African American folk medical system. The theory of humors focuses on the regulation of the body by the four humors, or major bodily fluids: blood, phlegm, black bile, and yellow bile. The liver, which produces bile, must be cleaned out every spring. Phlegm or mucus, often referred to as "slime," must be expelled from the body.

5. *Events, including illnesses, are attributed to phenomena that are classified as either "natural" or "unnatural."* Natural events are the result of phenomena that result from God's plan, thereby maintaining the balance or harmony of nature. Unnatural events are the result of phenomena created by the devil to upset or unbalance the harmony of nature. All negative events (including illnesses), whether they are natural or unnatural, can be rectified if their correct cause can be determined and means can be found to reestablish harmony with nature. The imbalance of natural events can be rectified by natural instruments and means such as physicians and biomedicine, but the imbalance of unnatural events can be set right only by supernatural approaches.

6. *The causes of natural illness.* The four major causes of natural illness are "cold," "dirt," improper diet, and improper conduct. Natural illnesses occur when a person fails to monitor or manipulate the bodily processes correctly. The body is then unprepared to defend itself against the forces of nature.

   a. *"Cold."* "Cold" is associated with an increase in the production of mucus, which results in the accumulation of phlegm in the kidneys or diaphragm. "Cold" enters the body when it is most vulnerable, and the elderly and very young are considered to be particularly susceptible. Illnesses that result from "cold" may not show up immediately; for instance, "cold" may enter the bodies of young people who do not take care of themselves and manifest itself only when they are older. Women are more susceptible to "cold" than men, especially during menstruation and right after childbirth, when bleeding causes the body to be "open." Because cold and dampness are thought to impede the flow of blood, women are warned not to wash their hair or do anything that may bring on a chill while bleeding. "Cold" can clot the blood, causing it to back up into the body. This may result in headache, stroke, and elevated blood pressure.

   b. *"Dirt."* "Dirt," vaguely associated with germs, is believed to circulate in the system via the blood. It may result from failure to bathe, impeded menses, irregular menses, or sexual excesses. Heat, fever, inflammation, and skin eruptions (including a baby's rash, measles, a syphilitic chancre, and skin cancer) are indications that something in the body is trying to come out.

Home remedies for "dirt." The idea of expelling "dirt" manifests itself in several ways, including an overconcern with the gastrointestinal tract. Many African Americans use, and overuse, laxatives, beginning in infancy. In the spring, many adults take additional laxatives to clean out the body. This treatment may consist of a nine-day course of sulfur and molasses to purify the body, castor oil to lubricate it, some form of commercial preparation to cleanse the liver, sassafras tea or poke greens to thin the blood (which is thought to thicken in winter), and numerous other cleansing treatments. It is highly important for caregivers to encourage patient disclosure of home remedies because some are quite dangerous. In addition to overusing laxatives, some African Americans have been known to take kerosene, turpentine, mothballs, and carbon tetrachloride as oral self-medications.

"Dirt" and menses. Another aspect of the "dirt" notion is its linkage with menses. Because of the belief that the function of menstruation is to rid the body of "dirty" blood, some African American women carefully monitor their blood flow during menstruation and after childbirth. Failure to bleed (e.g., during pregnancy) or a reduction in bleeding (e.g., due to the use of oral contraceptives) may cause concern that bad blood is being stored in the body and may back up and thicken, possibly causing hemorrhage or death. For this reason, many African Americans are resistant to the use of oral contraceptives.

"Dirt" and the womb. Because the mother does not menstruate during pregnancy, the environment inside the womb is considered unclean. Newborns are often given catnip tea to cause the eruption of hives or small red bumps, which are regarded as a way for the child's body to throw off the "filth" of the uterine environment.

"Dirt" and geophagy. Finally, another "dirt"-related phenomenon is *geophagy*, the eating of clay and dirt, a practice brought by slaves from Africa and considered to be particularly beneficial to pregnant women and their unborn children. Eating clay, which is rich in iron, may be both a cause and a result of anemia. With the end of slavery, when many African Americans moved from farming communities to towns and cities, Argo cornstarch was substituted for clay. Many older African Americans who acquired a taste for Argo years ago still eat it today.

c. *Improper diet (and its relation to "blood").* In the African American folk medical system, both the volume of blood and its distribution throughout the system are often dependent upon diet. African Americans often treat these folk illnesses, which are attributed to "high" or "low" blood, with home remedies and temporary changes in diet.

The condition referred to as "high blood" is associated with overly rich food and reddish foods, such as beets, carrots, grape juice, red wine, red meat, and pork. A diet rich in these foods is believed to send an oversupply of blood to the heart or brain, raising "pressure" and clogging these organs. Symptoms of "high blood" include "falling out" (sudden collapse in which the eyes usually remain open but the person cannot see), headache, dizziness, and spots before the eyes.

Natural remedies focus on lowering the blood "pressure" and thinning it out, opening the pores and sweating it out, and opening the bowels to eliminate pressure. Treatments include foods (many of them white in color), herbal teas, and laxatives. Remedies used in rural southern areas (where "high blood" may also be called "sweet blood") include "bitters," such as bullfrog urine mixed with garlic and onion. In urban areas, astringents such as vinegar, lemon juice, olive or pickle juice, garlic, and Epsom salts are common home remedies.

"Low blood" is associated with anemia; its symptoms are weakness, lassitude, and fatigue. It is home-treated with iron pills and tonic. The terms "high blood" and "low blood," which are widely used among African Americans, may lead to confusion of these folk terms with the medical conditions of high and low blood pressure. African American patients diagnosed with high or low blood pressure and given a long-term management plan may be reluctant to take medication indefinitely, fearing that too much high blood pressure medication may thin the blood and cause "low blood," and vice versa. Caregivers must take pains to explain carefully high or low blood pressure and the function of the prescribed medication. Patients may need to be reassured that long-term medication is necessary and will not result in the opposite condition.

d. *Improper conduct.* Because religion is an important component in the health/illness beliefs of many African Americans, disorders—especially in children—may be attributed to parents' transgressions and may need to be healed through prayer. For example, deformity, seizure disorders, and retardation in children may be interpreted as divine punishments for the parents' misdeeds. Home remedies and the ministrations of a physician alike are considered powerless in curing someone who has been punished by God. Only repentance through a contact with God, directly or through the intercession of a faith healer, can effect a cure.

7. *Unnatural illnesses and their causes, symptoms, and cures.* Unnatural (magical) illnesses are believed to be outside the realm of nature and unreachable by approaches that might be effective for natural illnesses. Successful treatment requires the intervention of a specialist who commands supernatural powers.

   Causes of unnatural illnesses. Unnatural illnesses may be caused by "worriation," evil influences, or sorcery. "Worriation" is produced by everyday stresses or concerns about daily problems. Evil influences result from God's withdrawal of protection from a person who has failed to mend his or her ways. Sorcery—or voodoo or rootwork—may "cross up," "fix," or "hex" someone. More often than not, the person responsible for the hex is someone inside the victim's social circle who intends harm because of anger, jealousy, or envy.

   Symptoms. Certain symptoms—nausea, vomiting, diarrhea, abdominal pain, lack of appetite, or loss of weight—may be interpreted as having been caused by sorcery, especially if someone cursed the victim or the victim has a guilty conscience. The means used by the sorcerer may be a magical poison, affecting only the intended victim, that was slipped into the person's food or drink.

   The sudden inability to perform daily tasks or the onset of erratic behavior may be attributed to a hex. A 1972 study conducted at a Miami psychiatric center found that one-third of all African American patients being treated for depression believed they were the victim of a hex.

   Patients who believe in sorcery may be very wary of eating anything outside the home or anything that they themselves have not prepared, convinced that the person who cast the spell on them can introduce such creatures as snakes, lizards, spiders, toads, or frogs into the victim's body by hiding their eggs or pulverized remains in food or drink.

   Cures. Only a powerful healer with supernatural powers can put on or take off a hex. Other folk healers will be powerless, as will physicians of biomedicine. It is even believed that the more the victim of an unnatural illness goes to a doctor, the sicker she or he will get. Often a person who believes she or he is hexed will try a biomedical cure first both as a way of confirming the existence of a hex and as a means of "testing" the physician's diagnostic ability and the "power" of her or his medicine.

Patients will most often withhold telling the caregiver of their suspicion of a hex (or even the fact that they believe in hexes) out of fear of ridicule.

Folk Healers among African American Populations

Many types of healers are found in African American communities. Some—such as the granny or herb doctor—work in their homes, while others practice in a religious setting. Some work on a one-to-one basis, and others in a group. Some healers claim to heal everything, while others confine themselves to a specific type of illness or problem. Whether they refer to themselves as healers, herb doctors, root doctors or root workers, readers, advisors, spiritualists, or conjurors, all claim that their healing power is a gift from God. They rarely refer to themselves as "Doctor," preferring kinship terms such as Sister, Brother, Mother, Reverend, Prophet, Evangelist, Madam, Princess, King, or Queen. Folk healers may advertise in local, community newspapers, in spite of the fact that they can be arrested for practicing medicine without a license.

Grannies, herbalists, and physicians. Healers are classified according to the origin of their healing power. Those who received their power through learning, such as the granny, herbalist, and medical physician, have the lowest status because of the belief that anyone may learn a healing trade. These healers are only allowed to treat natural illnesses.

Spiritual healers. Higher in status are those who received their gift during a profound religious experience; these are likely to be ministers who heal during regular church services that involve prayer, laying on of hands, and the use of holy oil or holy water with supernatural powers. Spiritual healers are believed to be successful in treating natural illnesses that have not responded to other forms of natural treatment and that may have been caused by sinning.

Supernatural healers. These are the healers of highest status, generally called sorcerers, voodooists, or root doctors, who are allowed to treat unnatural (magical) illnesses. Male voodoo healers are also called *houngan* or *papaloi,* while female healers are *mambo* or *mamaloi.* The most powerful supernatural healers are those believed to have been selected by God at birth. The seventh child of the same sex, the first child born after twins, and any child born with "the Vail" or caul (amniotic membrane) are likely to have been chosen. These healers are often treated with deference from birth and many have practiced healing since childhood. Reports of the details of voodoo healing rituals are sparse, but one of the most important involves the reading of animal bones. The bones (the source animal appears to be unimportant) are linked to physical attributes or body parts; the patient arranges the bones on the floor and the healer interprets the arrangement.

Identifying Patients Who May Have Used Folk Healing Methods

Fearing ridicule, patients who make use of folk healing methods will probably not admit it to the caregiver. When taking the initial history or performing a physical examination, the caregiver should gently probe the patient about the causes of the illness (which may reveal folk beliefs) and any treatments or remedies that have been tried. It is essential to listen closely and to avoid appearing judgmental or skeptical. If the patient admits to taking something that is not harmful, it is best to recommend its continued use. If, on the other hand, the patient reports taking something harmful, it is best to recommend against using it since it may clash with the powerful treatment that the caregiver will provide.

Another indicator of belief in folk medicine is the wearing of charms or amulets. These may include a silver dime (believed to turn black if someone is threatening harm); an amulet of asafetida, a strong-smelling plant gum resin, around the neck (believed to protect against contagious diseases); and copper or silver wrist bracelets (believed to provide early warning of illness by turning the skin around them black).

Helping "Hexed" Patients

If careful, sympathetic questioning reveals that the patient believes that he or she is the victim of a hex, the caregiver may take several approaches. One approach is to suggest hypnosis, during which the patient is reinforced in the belief that he or she is strong enough to throw off the hex. Another approach is to enter the patient's belief system by discussing the proposed treatment and suggesting that the patient consider it a more powerful "counter-hex." One physician went so far in the treatment of a patient with seizures as to stage a midnight healing ceremony, complete with candles, for the administration of intravenous medication, which was referred to as the most powerful anti-root medicine known. During the day, this information was reinforced by the nursing staff. The treatment worked; in ten days the patient was discharged from the hospital, feeling like his "old self."

This approach may or may not appear appropriate. The caregiver must use judgment to avoid patronizing or misinforming the patient, but it may be possible to partner with the patient in attacking a hex "on its own terms." In the face of the patient's belief that the physician will be powerless against a hex, an unconventional approach might be justified to convince the patient that modern biomedicine can help. It has now become more common for hospitals and clinics to work with *curanderos* for Latino patients who believe in folk medicine. It may be possible to make similar arrangements with voodoo healers.

DEVELOPING CULTURAL PERSPECTIVE

1. Upon being diagnosed with a chronic illness, what belief system might cause an African American to search for another caregiver or another diagnosis?

2. In dark-skinned individuals, why may a blood test be needed to confirm the presence of jaundice?

3. In dark-skinned individuals, is pallor defined as the absence of white skin tones or red skin tones?

4. Why might washing one's hair during menstruation or during an illness be contraindicated by a patient's belief system?

5. When would recommending eating more beets and carrots for someone with high blood pressure be contraindicated by a patient's belief system?

6. Why might the patient's family interpret the sudden inability of the patient to perform daily tasks as a spiritual problem and not a medical problem?

BLENDING PERSPECTIVES

1. Can a healthcare practitioner who treats only the symptoms deliver "effective" healthcare to a patient who believes that illness manifests when the balance of body, mind, and soul is disturbed?

2. How can the question, "What medicines, vitamins, or herbs are you currently taking?" be revised to encompass home remedies such as liver cleansers, eating clay, or eating cornstarch?

Chapter 3

Providing Culture-Sensitive Healthcare to American Indians and Alaska Natives

Keys to a Good Professional Relationship with American Indian and Alaska Native Patients

1. *Make the patient welcome.* First meetings are important! To make the patient feel welcome, extend a warm greeting and smile. The smile may not be returned, but it will be appreciated. Shake hands, introduce yourself, and allow the patient to do the same (thereby showing respect to his or her ancestors). Thank the patient for having chosen your health facility. Although a Western-style handshake is appropriate and appreciated, don't be surprised if it is returned by an unusually weak one. The traditional Navajo greeting is not to shake hands, but to extend the hand and gently touch the other person's hand.

2. *Use eye contact judiciously.* Although eye contact is expected during the initial handshake and occasionally during the interview, prolonged eye contact is considered a sign of disrespect and should be avoided.

3. *Accommodate tribal healing.* Patients may wish to perform certain tribal healing ceremonies, perhaps, even in the hospital (e.g., sprinkling corn or cornmeal around the bed before surgery or treatment, burying the umbilical cord after childbirth). Try to accommodate these ceremonies as a means of improving both the patient's and the family's confidence in the care.

4. *Show special respect to the elderly.* Great respect is given to the elderly, in spite of taboos connected with death. Caregivers gain approval by treating the elderly with kindness and respect and not appearing to criticize or scold them.

5. *Think carefully about family care.* Poverty, distance from the medical facility, and taboos against dying in the home may make it impractical to release a patient needing long-term or terminal care to the family. Discuss options with the family and try to ascertain their attitudes about caring for the person at home.

6. *Involve the extended family.* The extended family plays an important role in healthcare decision making. Often many family members will appear with a patient who is to be admitted for a hospital stay. Try to arrange a place for them to wait or to stay for a longer period as close as possible to the patient

and the hospital. Include family members when decisions regarding treatment options are needed. Very often, a patient will postpone surgery because the consent of the family leader, often the eldest female, must be obtained first.

7. *Appreciate a different sense of time.* American Indians and Alaska Natives tend to be present-oriented. Traditionally time is viewed as a continuum with no beginning and no end. This concept can cause difficulty in organizing future events, such as the regulation of medication. Caregivers should be wary of telling patients to take medications with meals, as the patient may have three meals today, two meals tomorrow, and four meals the day after that. In addition, many American Indians and Alaska Natives are task-conscious rather than time-conscious, paying more to the needs of the task than to finishing it within a set period of time or sticking to an appointment schedule. If possible, ask the patient for help in linking appointments or medication schedules to events that are certain to happen in the patient's daily life.

8. *Give and expect generosity.* American Indian culture discourages competitive behavior and encourages giving, sharing, and cooperation. Generosity and doing things for others are regarded highly.

9. *Take your time.* It is important to spend time with patients and to avoid appearing hurried or nervous. Patients often travel great distances at great financial hardship to see a physician. It sends a negative message if the physician spends only five or ten minutes with them.

10. *Speak plainly.* During an examination, avoid medical or other terms that may not be understood, but at the same time, don't talk down to the patient or appear to treat him or her as a child. A soft, concerned voice will do much to make the patient feel at ease.

11. *Respect silence.* Be concise and give the patient time to reflect on what you are saying. Don't try to fill up the time. American Indians are taught the value of silence and may also need time to mentally translate what they hear into their own language.

12. *Understand tribal diagnosis.* Traditional and scientific medicines are not mutually exclusive, so the patient may have come to you after having been seen by a tribal healer. The patient may be unfamiliar with the biomedical approach of identifying the specific location of pain because tribal healers use different procedures. It is, therefore, sometimes more helpful to ask the patient to point to the most intense area of pain rather than asking, "Where is the pain?" and expecting a verbal reply.

Health Problems and Concerns Common to American Indians and Alaska Natives

1. *Shorter life expectancy.* The average life expectancy for American Indians and Alaska Natives is 71.1 and 70.6 years, respectively, compared to 76.5 years for other races in the United States. Infant mortality is also greater, with 8.9 deaths per every 1,000 live births as compared to 7.2 per 1,000 for all other races.

   According to the Indian Health Service of the U.S. Department of Health and Human Services, the five leading causes of death among American Indians from 1994 to 1996 were: (1) heart disease, (2) malignant neoplasms, (3) accidents, (4) diabetes mellitus, and (5) chronic liver disease. Other major causes of death are (6) pneumonia and (7) influenza, (8) homicide, (9) suicide, and (10) chronicobstructive pulmonary disease. Many health problems and the high incidence of accidents and suicides may be due, in part, either directly or indirectly to poverty, feelings of hopelessness, and adjustment problems.

2. *High infant death rate.* This can be attributed to a high incidence of diarrhea, a harsh physical environment, and the failure of many women to seek prenatal care. Because pregnancy and birth are considered natural and normal processes on the one hand, and healthcare facilities are associated with illness and disease on the other, many Indian women do not seek prenatal care.

3. *Strict separation of pregnancy and disease.* Pregnant Navajo women, for example, are forbidden to attend traditional healing ceremonies to avoid contact with illness or disease. For this reason, one researcher advises holding maternal and child care clinics in a location separate from other clinical services.

4. *Type 2 diabetes.* According to the Indian Health Service, American Indians and Alaska Natives have the highest prevalence of type 2 diabetes in the world. This high incidence of non-insulin-dependent diabetes has increased dramatically since 1940 even among those in their teens and early twenties. American Indians have a genetic predisposition to diabetes that has now been triggered by a radical change in eating habits and increase in obesity resulting from military service during World War II. The military experience, with its exposure to different groups and its comparatively high pay, produced a drastic change in dietary habits and lifestyle. High-cholesterol fast foods began to replace the traditional diet.

    Among the Sioux, Chippewa, Pueblo, and Cherokee, about one-third of adults over age 35 have type 2 diabetes. The incidence among the Pima—about one-half the population—is the highest in the world. The prevalence of diabetes among the Ute Indians is 4 times the national average, and the rate of diabetic neuropathy 43 times that of the non-Ute population in Utah. Complications such as amputations occur at a rate 2 to 3 times, and renal failure at a rate about 20 times, that of the general population. The Indian Health Service is trying to combat diabetes through education, including classes in cooking and nutrition. One important ally in these attempts has been the traditional belief in a harmony of body, mind, and spirit.

    In an effort to curb diabetes in American Indians and Alaska Natives, the Centers for Disease Control and Prevention have now developed a regional training program called "Diabetes Today." This program offers training in community-based planning to treat diabetes in culturally appropriate ways. The Association of American Indian Physicians and the National Diabetes Education Program American Indian/Alaska Native Work Group have also developed school programs aimed at diabetes prevention among American Indian and Alaska Native youth. Information about these programs can be found at *www.aaip.com/diabetes/diabetes.html.*

5. *Tuberculosis.* The incidence of tuberculosis among some Indian peoples is high, ranging from 2 percent among the Apache to 4.6 percent among the Navajo. This may be largely due to socioeconomic factors, such as overcrowding and poor nutrition.

6. *Myocardial infarction.* A 1988 study of myocardial infarction showed a considerable increase, compared with earlier studies, among Navajo men and a gradual increase among Navajo women. About 50 percent of those who suffered acute infarcts were hypertensive, and the other 50 percent were diabetic; 31 percent were both. Although hypertension is low among residents of reservations, it is common among Indians who live in urban areas.

7. *Alcoholism.* A fact sheet published by the American Indian Health Service in 2002 states that the death rate from alcoholism is 7 times higher for American Indians than for the rest of the population, and in 1997–99 alcoholism accounted for 47.0 deaths per 100,000 persons.

Although alcoholism is reported to be more significant in men than women, a recent pilot study of fetal alcohol syndrome (FAS) found FAS in 3.9 percent of live births. This figure may underestimate the true rate because (a) parents or guardians are reluctant to bring children suspected of FAS for evaluation, (b) some physicians don't diagnose possible alcohol-damaged children out of reluctance to label the child, and (c) many infants die before they are tested for FAS. Researchers studying FAS in the northern plains region urge a counseling and treatment program for all pregnant women who drink alcohol and more careful surveillance for FAS.

Alcohol has also been a contributing factor in a large percentage of motor vehicle deaths, homicides, and suicides.

8. *Pediatric health.* Navajo children have low length-for-age and high weight-for-length measures because of suboptimal nutrition. One study suggests that growth abnormalities among Navajo infants are the result of intrauterine growth retardation and low birth weight.

9. *Improper diet.* Of the 10 leading causes of death among American Indians, five are related to diet. Navajo classify foods in terms of strong and weak foods. Strong foods—for the most part, the nineteenth century reservation foods, such as mutton, game, and other animal foods; fried bread; Indian corn; and potatoes—are believed to promote health. Milk is the most frequently mentioned weak food. It is probably no coincidence that about 79 percent of American Indians are lactose intolerant. It is believed that it is all right for the elderly to drink goat's milk and for the infant to drink mother's milk, but milk, in general, is not considered a healthful food.

Traditional American Indian Care and Treatment

Care-seeking behaviors. A 1962 study of the healthcare decision-making process of 77 American Indians living close to an Indian Health Service (IHS) hospital found that 10 individuals (13%) elected not to seek care of any kind. Of the 67 persons who did seek care, 32 (48%) elected to seek modern medical care exclusively, 26 (39%) used both native healers and physicians, and only nine (13%) used Native practitioners exclusively.

In general, the more years of education, the more likely it is that an American Indian will have been raised off a reservation (only 43.8 percent of American Indians now live in rural areas served by the American Indian Health Service, while 56.2 percent live in urban areas) and the less likely it is that he or she will use traditional methods of healing. For those with less education, it is not uncommon to consult first a traditional healer to diagnose or remove the cause of a disease, and then visit an Indian Health Service physician. One researcher has pointed out that the Navajo practice of combining traditional ceremonies and biomedical services may result more from the inaccessibility of hospitals and clinics and the difficulty in communicating with caregivers than from a preference for traditional cures.

Home treatment. Economic factors, knowledge about and access to herbs, and distance from biomedical care often influence the decision to seek home treatment. However, as more over-the-counter remedies become available at trading posts and cash-and-carry stores, these remedies are becoming more popular than herbal remedies for a wide number of symptoms.

Traditional diagnosis, rituals, and ceremonies. When illness is perceived, a "hand trembler" or "stargazer" may be asked to diagnose the cause. He or she will use a trance, induced by a simple ritual, to "see" or "hear" the cause of the illness. A ceremonialist or "singer" may then be engaged to remove the illness through the appropriate healing ceremony. In Navajo culture, more than 75 different healing ceremonies have been identified. In addition, "blessing way" chants may also be performed as a way to prevent illness, maintain health, and attract the forces of beauty and harmony.

The healing ceremony should be performed four times to ensure the removal of the cause of illness, a requirement that involves a great deal of expense. Because most healing ceremonies are forbidden during summer months, there can be a long waiting period between diagnosis and cure. During these times, an herbalist is often engaged to relieve symptoms. However, it is becoming more and more common for people to self-diagnose simple illnesses or go to an Indian Health Service physician, where care is provided free of charge.

Navajo who live in close proximity to other tribal villages may sometimes use the traditional healers associated with those villages. Hopi healers, for example, are believed to be experts at healing through "sucking cures," which "suck" the intrusive, illness-causing object from the body. Peyote cures are also used.

American Indian Religious and Spiritual Beliefs That Can Affect Care and Treatment

In spite of the enormous diversity in tribal cultures, languages, and religious beliefs of the almost 300 American Indian tribes living within the continental United States, these tribes share a number of fundamental health, illness, and illness prevention beliefs such as:

1. Life comes from the Great Spirit (or Supreme Creator) and all healing begins with Him.
2. Man is a threefold being made up of body, mind, and spirit.
3. Health or wellness is due to a preservation of harmony among the body, heart, mind, and soul.
4. Plants and animals, as well as humans, are part of the spirit world that exists alongside, and is intermingled with, the physical world.
5. Death is not an enemy but a natural phenomenon of life.
6. The spirit existed before it came into a physical body and will exist after the body dies.
7. Spirituality and emotions are just as important as the body and the mind.
8. Our relationships with others and with the earth itself are an essential component of our health.
9. Illness affects the mind and spirit as well as the body.
10. Illness is an opportunity to purify one's soul.
11. Disease is felt not only by the individual, but also by the family.
12. Natural ill health is caused by the violation of a sacred tribal taboo; unnatural ill health is caused by witchcraft.
13. The individual is responsible for his or her own wellness.
14. Mother Earth provides numerous remedies for our illnesses.
15. Traditional healers can be either men or women, young or old.

THE NAVAJO TRIBE: AN EXAMPLE

The Navajo Application of These Beliefs

According to the 2000 U.S. Census, the Navajo tribe has about 250,000 members, the majority living on a reservation of about 27,000 square miles of semiarid land in Arizona, New Mexico, Utah, and Colorado. The information that follows illustrates how one important American Indian culture applies the general beliefs listed above to its health practices. Although the application of these beliefs may vary by tribe, it is hoped that the detailed description of Navajo beliefs will serve to improve the caregiver's understanding of how these beliefs may affect the health behavior of other tribal nations as well.

Navajo society is matriarchal, built on the belief that a goddess known as First Woman, Spirit Woman, Whiteshell Woman, Thinking Woman, or Changing Woman created the universe. In Navajo society, women hold a higher position than men. According to tribal custom, the husband moves into the home of the wife's parents upon marriage. The extended family, often called a "camp," generally comprises the senior married couple, their unmarried children, their married daughters, and the daughters' husbands. Traditional Navajo must obtain the permission of the leading female elder before entering a hospital or undergoing surgery.

A fundamental guiding principle of Navajo life is beauty, or *hozho*. *Hozho* encompasses not only the concept of beauty but also blessedness, goodness, order, and harmony. It defines the traditional Navajo way of thinking and relating to others and the world. The principle of *hozho* guides everyday thought, speech, and behavior, and shapes Navajo rituals and religious ceremonies. Traditional Navajo religion focuses on maintaining a harmonious relationship with all living things, including the land, one's farm, and one's community. Maintaining this harmonious relationship is essential to one's health; if one falls into disharmony, illness will result.

A person maintains his or her balance and harmony with nature by both actions and words. Reality mirrors the spoken word. Because words not only describe the world but also help create it, words must be chosen carefully.

As a rule, the Navajo may not seek medical care for a number of discomforts and acute illnesses for which a non-Navajo would most likely seek relief. Illness, like death, is simply viewed and accepted as a natural part of life.

Navajo Etiology Of Disease

The aim of Navajo healing ceremonies is to remove the cause of a disease, not just alleviate the symptoms. These ceremonies incorporate *hozho,* the spoken word, and the concept of *nayee,* or monsters from Navajo mythology used to conceptualize everything that keeps a person from life. These ceremonies can vary in nature from an hour-long prayer to nine days of singing and chanting. When a person approaches a healer, he simply states the problem, asks for assistance, and waits silently for instructions. The healer may use one of three traditional approaches to find the source of the disharmony: stargazing (looking at the stars either directly or through a crystal), listening to heard messages, or hand trembling. It is interesting to note that while the ceremonies seek to destroy the *nayee,* or monsters that keep the person from living his life, the monsters of Hunger, Old Age, Poverty, and Dirt are not destroyed because they are considered a necessary part of life.

The Causes of Disease Are Thought to Be:

Soul loss. The soul or "wind" of a person enters the body at birth, forming the basic personality. Until the baby laughs for the first time—an indication that the wind has attached itself to the body—it is believed that the baby may die easily. In old age, the soul is again loosely attached, making death natural. The ghosts of the very young and very old are not considered agents of disease, but if a person with well-attached wind dies, the ghost of that person is thought to be an extremely dangerous and potent agent of disease. Therefore, there is a general taboo against touching the dead—possibly due to uncertainty about whether the soul is still attached to the body and will be a disease agent.

Intrusive objects. In a special form of witchcraft called "wizardry," a disease-causing agent can be injected into the skin of the victim by a witch or sorcerer.

Spirit intrusion or possession. This happens when the spirit or "wind" of an individual is displaced by the spirit of a dangerous supernatural being.

Breach of taboo. The most frequent diagnosis of illness is linked with various taboos. A person who goes into general seizures is suspected of incest. This illness is frequently called "moth sickness," in reference to the mythical butterfly people who committed the first incest. Because the moth is the etiological agent and the disease may result from contact with it, a witch can cause this illness by making a person touch a real moth.

Witchcraft or sorcery. A witch is defined as a person who has killed someone, generally a relative, and then changed himself or herself into an animal (such as a wolf, coyote, bear, owl, fox, dog, crow, eagle, porcupine, snake, moth, or long-horned grasshopper) in order to travel and do evil undetected. Witches band together for rituals and ceremonies involving chants, sand paintings, body paintings, and masks. They are believed to perform their witchery by touching the victim with a powder made from a bit of the flesh of the dead. Signs of having been the victim of witchery are fainting and unconsciousness. Another sort of witchcraft, called "frenzy witchcraft," is associated primarily with love magic. This witchcraft uses various plant species of the *Datura* genus, which contain scopolamine and hyoscyamine; when ingested, they can produce hallucinations, dissociative reactions, and even coma. It is believed that a mere touch of the potion can cause a woman to tear off her clothes in a sexual frenzy, permitting the witch to seduce her.

Sorcery is only slightly different from witchery. Sorcerers cast spells on people in absentia by using bits of the person's hair, nails, feces, or other body products.

Combined Use of Traditional and Modern Medicine

A Navajo would probably not question the value of using both "modern" medicine and Navajo medicine. The two approaches to health and illness are viewed as distinct but complementary. It is perfectly acceptable for a person to consult a Navajo diagnostician to identify the cause of a disease and to arrange a ceremony to eliminate the cause, as well as to consult a physician to alleviate the symptoms of the disease. Similarly, it is not uncommon for some Navajo to insist that they be allowed to hold a traditional ceremony or ritual before undergoing surgery or treatment at a reservation hospital. An important difference is that, whereas a traditional diagnostician or healer may advise the ill person to seek treatment from a physician, the reverse is rarely the case.

Navajo Language and the Classification of Illness

Illnesses are classified by the agents believed to have caused them or the ceremonies used to cure them—such as the Wind Way, the Evil Way, the Night Way, the Plume Way, and the Earth and Beauty Way—rather than by either the symptoms expressed or the parts of the body affected. Since diagnosis does not rely on an understanding of symptoms, many traditional Navajo may be confused by the physician's need to ask questions while taking a medical history or conducting a physical examination. However, studies indicate that the ability to describe the nuances of pain and symptoms in the Navajo language is highly sophisticated and that patients can become good historians of their illnesses if they are helped to understand why the physician needs a good history.

Peyote Religion and Its Impact on Navajo Health Beliefs and Practices

Full traditional ceremonies and rituals—which may last from five to nine nights and often involve hosting large numbers of guests—are becoming increasingly infrequent. The number of qualified medicine men and women has also declined, largely because as many as eight years of training and apprenticeship are needed to learn each major ceremony. Most ceremonialists, therefore, limit themselves to the performance of only two of these major ceremonies.

The Peyote religion, now organized as the Native American Church, offers a simpler and more economical way to hold ceremonies. Peyote is a nativistic religion that began among the Kiowa and Comanche tribes during the second half of the nineteenth century. The Peyote religion has achieved ready acceptance among the Navajo because it neither introduces new beliefs about the causes of disease nor denies any beliefs central to Navajo religion. Its short, one-night ceremonies, performed on weekends, offer a practical substitute for long and expensive Navajo healing ceremonies, especially for working Navajo who cannot afford to take off from work to attend ceremonies that can last as long as a week or even more.

Because Peyote ceremonies are not only short but also easy to learn, Navajo youth who wish to gain status through traditional means can easily become Peyote healers. For similar reasons, the number of American Indians who have joined and become active in fundamentalist Christian denominations, such as the Nazarene, Pentecostal, and Baptist religions, has increased.

Combined Use of Peyote Ceremonies and Other Medical Systems to Relieve Symptoms

However, in spite of the fact that the Navajo use Peyote ceremonies, healers from the neighboring Hopi and other tribes, faith healers, Christian ministers, and practitioners of modern medicine, these new approaches have not really become an integral part of the Navajo belief system. This system is sacred and lies at the core of Navajo religion. The fact that many Navajo use other medical systems does not signify any real, underlying change in their understanding of health prevention, health maintenance, or cure, because, as stated earlier, these newer medical approaches relieve symptoms, rather than removing the cause of the disease.

DEVELOPING CULTURAL PERSPECTIVE

1. Why might a hospital's normal visiting hours and limitations for visitors be constraining for an American Indian?

2. Many medications have components in common with plants (example: fever-few has acetylsalicyclic acid, the basis for aspirin). How would explaining similarities between a medication and a naturally occurring substance enhance compliance for an American Indian?

3. How might eye contact be modified to make an American Indian or Alaska Native feel more comfortable?

BLENDING PERSPECTIVES

1. How can patient privacy be safeguarded within a culture that values group collaboration, sharing, and group decision-making?

2. In a system that demands tight patient schedules, how might staff seek to accommodate a patient whose interpretation of being "on time" for an appointment varies from the norm?

Providing Culture-Sensitive Healthcare to Patients of Asian Origin

Keys to a Good Professional Relationship with Asian Patients

It is important to keep in mind that the term "Asian" is very general and may be used to identify the many population groups (totaling more than half the world's population) who originate from the world's largest continent. In practice, the term is used to denote groups from East Asia and Southeast Asia, such as Chinese, Japanese, Koreans, Vietnamese, Thai, Laotians, Hmong, and Cambodians. The cultures of these groups, although quite distinct from one another, share many common threads due to a history of Chinese influence that includes ties to Buddhist and Confucian thought and religion. This group will be broadly referred to as "Asians" in this text, to be distinguished from South Asians, who are from India, Pakistan, Bangladesh, and Sri Lanka. Some additional information is provided about the almost 200,000 Hmong people living in the United States because, although most come from the mountainous regions of northern Laos, their isolation from other Asians has led to the development of some very distinct cultural and health beliefs and practices. Lack of knowledge about Hmong history, culture, and health beliefs has resulted in problems in delivery of healthcare to this population. Although the Philippines is geographically part of Southeast Asia, Filipino culture is also discussed separately because its history has been heavily influenced by Spanish culture, which has led to distinct differences from other Asian cultural groups.

The suggestions below should be considered only very general guidelines. While there are enough common social practices and rules of etiquette within the Asian community for the following suggestions to prove helpful when working with most Asian patients, the distinctions mentioned above should be kept in mind. Furthermore, such factors as specific country of origin or ancestry, length of stay in the United States, age, living environment, educational level, and socioeconomic status will play an important part in determining each individual's needs and expectations. These guidelines should provide a practical starting point for establishing a good relationship with members of this large and diverse group.

1. *Follow general Asian rules of etiquette.* Asian societies tend to be highly stratified by age and social structure. Caregivers should understand and observe rules of social interaction, such as the following:

a. Greet elders first and address them in a formal manner. Since physicians hold a very high position in Asian society, the patient may show respect to even a young physician by looking away when talking to avoid meeting the physician's eye.

b. Do not sit with your legs crossed, lean on a table or desk, or point at anything with your foot when talking. These behaviors are all considered signs of contempt toward the person one is addressing.

2. *Be aware of forms of greeting and address.* Chinese, Japanese, and Koreans address one another by surname (which may be given first when the patient is asked for his or her name). They tend to address family members in terms of position in the family (e.g., Older Brother, Mother, Eldest Daughter, Middle Son, Husband). Long-term close friends may address one another by the family name followed by an honorific, such as *san* in Japanese. Southeast Asians are more at ease if they are addressed by their first names and greeted warmly, and if the caregiver shows a personal interest in their lives and families. One Laotian interviewee suggests that trinkets be kept on hand as token gifts to patients with children.

3. *Understand the importance of the head and the blood.* Many Asian cultures consider the head the most sacred part of a human being, so the caregiver should never touch or reach over it without first obtaining the person's—or parent's—permission to do so. If a caregiver pats a child on the head or rumples the child's hair, and then the child becomes ill, the physician may be blamed for taking the child's soul and causing the illness.

Since many Asians view blood as a vital element, in traditional Asian medicine blood is not drawn for medical purposes. In fact, some Asians believe that venipuncture not only upsets the body's natural balance but weakens the person, because the body does not replenish lost blood. Caregivers should exercise restraint in the number of tests they order that involve drawing blood. When blood must be drawn, the patient should be assured that only small amounts will be drawn and that the blood will not be given to anyone else. Blood is believed to represent a person's essence and the thought that one's essence may be given to someone else can cause great fear.

4. *Understand possible views of dosages and oral medications.* Although it is traditional to expect doctors to prescribe medication (or, at the very least, recommend changes in diet), some patients may adjust the dosage downward—to as little as a half-dose—because they consider most Western or biomedical medicines "hot" and overly potent—especially to Asians, who tend to be smaller in stature than Westerners. The patient may even discontinue the medication completely without consulting the physician if the symptoms are no longer present or if there has been no relief of the symptoms within a few days.

Many Chinese are not familiar with taking pills. Chinese medication is more often steeped in water and drunk in the form of a tea or as a slush. Southeast Asian patients, on the other hand, tend to believe that medication in the form of an injection is more effective than oral medication.

5. *Understand how harmony and "face" may mask noncompliance.* Although some Asian patients may appear to understand a diagnosis and accept a treatment plan, they may fail to comply. Noncompliance may be attributable to the concepts of harmony and "face." Because of a cultural respect for harmony, Asian patients who don't understand a treatment or even disagree with it may avoid conflict and suppress negative thoughts and emotions. This is because nonacceptance of a request, especially if that request is made by a physician, would disrupt harmony. Further, to maintain both their "face" and the physician's, some Asian patients may avoid admitting that they don't understand the diagnosis or treatment plan, or may even pretend to accept it when in fact

they do not. Caregivers should learn to observe the indirect (often nonverbal) signs that indicate confusion or displeasure about the diagnosis or treatment plan and should "test" their patients' comprehension. Rather than ask an Asian patient "Do you understand the diagnosis/treatment?" it is better to ask the patient to describe the condition or to describe what he or she has been told to do in his or her own words.

6. *Adjust schedules to accommodate holidays.* At the time of Asian holidays, it may not be effective to schedule medical appointments or procedures. Regular dietary, sleeping, and eating patterns may be interrupted. Women especially are preoccupied with cleaning and food preparation. No one wants to think about illness or medical problems.

Fundamental Health Concepts of East Asians and Southeast Asians

Yin and yang. Traditionally most groups from Asia define health as the harmonious balance between the forces of *yin* and *yang* and the corresponding conditions of "hot" and "cold." Illness is attributed to an upset of this balance. Illness can be cured only if the balance is restored by lowering the excessive trait or increasing the deficient one. Most traditional medical investigation involves a search for imbalances within the patient's physical and mental self. Treatment focuses on the restoration of balance.

"Hot" and "cold" theory of disease. Everything in the universe is classified as either *yin*, which is "cold," or *yang*, which is "hot." The terms refer not to temperatures but to attributes and/or conditions based upon *yin* and *yang*. The "hot"/"cold" classification, which is applied as much to recently discovered diseases and biomedical treatments as to traditional ones, includes parts of the body and their functions (e.g., childbirth), diseases, foods, and medicines. A "hot" disease is treated by a "cold" medicine in order to rebalance the patient's condition. Linden tea, for example, which may be served hot, is considered a "cold" herb and is used to treat "hot" ailments. Penicillin, on the other hand, is considered a "hot" treatment because it can produce diarrhea and rashes, which are viewed as "hot" symptoms.

While not all Asian patients subscribe to these beliefs, no caregiver can afford to ignore the possibility that a particular patient may be influenced consciously or unconsciously by them to some degree. Their effect on both trust and adherence to prescribed treatments can be enormous. For example, water and fruit juice are "cold" substances that are to be avoided during illness and after childbirth, times that produce a "cold" condition. Consequently, Asian patients may greatly curtail their fluid intake and may be reluctant to bathe or shower for as long as 30 days, since water conducts "cold" into the body. If a Western-trained physician prescribes cold liquids to a person with a cold who is running a high fever, not only might the patient ignore the physician's advice, but also he or she might question the medical knowledge of the physician.

Qi or Ch'i. Other important traditional Asian concepts about healthcare are blood and an energy force known in Chinese as *Qi,* sometimes written and pronounced in English as *Ch'i.* The generation and flow of blood through the vessels and the flow of the energy force (*Qi*) through the meridians or acupuncture points are the fundamental factors most involved in the harmonious/disharmonious states of the body. Blood is believed to be "ruled by the heart, governed by the spleen, and stored in the liver." *Qi* involves all organs, but has a special relationship with the liver, lungs, and spleen. When the flow of *Qi* is blocked by a broken bone or disease, acupuncture at the meridians permits the force to flow freely again.

Asian Dietary Beliefs and Practices That Affect Healthcare

Harmony. Diet plays a major role in Asian health and illness beliefs and many preventives and cures depend on regulating or changing the diet. Because foods and beverages are classified as either *yin* or *yang,* "cold" or "hot," what one eats has a major influence on the balance and harmony essential to health. Many Asian groups, such as the Chinese, Japanese, and Koreans, believe that their cuisine naturally balances these forces. To some extent, this may be true. For example, a study of the symptoms of menopause among women in rural Japan and women in the West found fewer menopausal symptoms among the Japanese women, a finding attributed to a Japanese diet high in soybean, a substance that contains natural estrogen.

Hospital food and its conflict with Asian diet. Many aspects of the Western diet, which are reflected in dietary suggestions made by physicians and by the food served in hospitals, conflict with beliefs about the balance of "hot" and "cold." In addition, many Asians are lactose intolerant. Salads and raw vegetables are also strange to people who derive most of their vegetable nutrients from stir-frying. Because an Asian patient may find hospital food strange and unappealing, it is customary for relatives to bring food from home. In most cases, the food will provide the patient with a healthful, balanced meal with which he or she is familiar, and hospital staff should be counseled to accept this custom.

Asian "chicken soup." Rice soup with chicken is a common "illness food" among Southeast Asians. It is also believed to diminish the severity of scars from surgery.

Beef and eggs. Many Southeast Asians believe that neither beef nor eggs should be served to those who are ill.

Childbirth. After childbirth Asian women prefer to eat mostly fish and avoid deep-fried foods, meats in any form of sauce, and spicy foods.

The role of the wife or mother. Since the wife or mother is firmly in charge of the Asian family kitchen, any recommended change of diet for her family members should be discussed with her.

"Mix and Match" Approach to Care

In general, most Asians do not seem to perceive any great dichotomy between the Eastern and Western medical belief systems. There is a widespread belief that some illnesses are best treated by traditional medicine (with roots primarily in Chinese medicine) and others by Western physicians. For example, Western physicians are often consulted for problems involving dentistry, fever, allergy, eye problems, heart attack, stroke, surgery, diabetes, and cancer, while traditional physicians and herbalists are sought for asthma, arthritis, bruises, sprains, lumbago, stomach problems, and hypertension.

Often a Western physician is visited for diagnosis and treatment, but, once the complaint has been diagnosed, the person will self-medicate by using herbs and patent medicines purchased over the counter. If the Western treatment doesn't bring immediate relief of the symptoms, the patient may seek the care of a traditional physician or healer. The same thing may happen if a Western diagnosis is rejected because it bears a negative prognosis (including diagnosis of a long-term illness or of an illness that cannot be fully cured) or because surgery is advised. The traditional treatment may either replace the Western treatment or be used along with it. Many Asian patients do not disclose the use of traditional care and medications to their Western physicians because the two medical domains—Western and traditional medicine—are seen as entirely separate. Some patients may also fear that the Western physician (an authority figure) will disapprove, or they believe that disclosure of the traditional care would violate the relationship of trust.

Asian Medical Treatments That May Be Used as Alternatives or Additions to Western Care

Most traditional medical interventions that may be sought by Asian patients living in America are versions of healing practices that originated in China and then spread throughout Asia.

Acupuncture. This treatment, which is also becoming more popular with Westerners, was developed by Chinese physicians between 106 B.C.E. and 220 C.E. Its purpose is to treat an excess of *yang* and restore the balance between *yin* and *yang.* It involves the application of nine needles to specific meridian points in the body. These meridians are said to extend to a fixed network of 360 points where the lines emerge.

Treatments wrongly interpreted as abuse. Three Asian medical treatments that leave welts difficult to distinguish from the bruises left by beatings have been the source of much misunderstanding between Asian parents who have recently immigrated to the West and Western educators and social workers who come into contact with their children. Many parents whose children have been administered these treatments by family members or healers have been charged with child abuse and have had their children taken from them. The marks of these treatments have also led to investigations of spousal abuse when unknowing caregivers have observed them on female patients.

Coining and pinching. This is a treatment in which a metal coin is dipped in oil, heated, and then rubbed briskly over the skin until welts appear. These welts can also be produced by pinching the skin between the thumb and index finger. These procedures are used as a means of drawing out fever and illness. This procedure leaves long lines of continuous dark bruises over the skin.

Cupping. This treatment involves suction produced by heating and applying small tubes or hot cups to the forehead or abdomen. The cups produce a negative pressure as they cool, resulting in a circular ecchymosis on the skin.

Moxibustion. This treatment for an excess of *yin* ("cold") is based upon a notion of the therapeutic value of heat. Pulverized wormwood or other burning incense is heated and applied to the torso, head, or neck to produce superficial burns. Sometimes this treatment accompanies acupuncture.

Herbs. Herbs, in the form of a slush, tea, or other drink, are an important part of traditional medicine in all Asian cultures. Herbal remedies require prescriptions from traditional healers. These remedies can be very expensive.

Home remedies. Many Asians routinely engage in home preventive treatment. Sometimes the treatment consists of nothing more than the use of cooling drinks and foods in hot weather and heating foods and drinks in cold weather. Asians often find other curative treatments, such as tonics and herbs and changes in diet, by consulting family and friends or by reading home medical manuals that list home remedies. These herbs and patent medicines, which can be purchased over the counter in herbal dispensaries or groceries, are often a person's first recourse at the initial sign of illness, before any form of medical help is sought. With home remedies, as with medical care, "mixing and matching" and "trial and error" are very common. Patients may buy two or three patent medicines with the same ingredients, or patent medicines that duplicate herbal prescriptions, to test their effectiveness. They may also take herbal medications in combination with prescriptions from Western physicians or even experiment with the dosages prescribed by physicians.

Systems of Religious Thought That Affect Health Beliefs and Practices: Confucian, Buddhist, and Taoist "Threads That Bind"

The similarities in social structure, communication style, and healthcare beliefs and practices that link very diverse groups of East Asian and Southeast Asian Americans can be traced to the interrelated and overlapping philosophical and religious teachings of Confucianism, Buddhism, and Taoism. These beliefs, including the concepts of *yin* and *yang*, the five elements, harmony, *tao* (the "way"), the golden mean, and nature and fate, originated in China and then radiated outward to Japan, Korea, Southeast Asia, and the Philippines.

Ancestor worship. Ancestor worship is an important link in the Asian religious and belief system, as well as in attitudes about health, illness, and forms of cure. The brightly colored altars with offerings of fruit and flowers (and sometimes even articles of clothing) that Westerners are apt to notice when entering an Asian home or place of business honor the family's ancestors, who are often asked to watch over members of the family and prevent or cure illness.

Yin and yang. Even older than the religious philosophies described above is the cosmological principle of complementary duality, better known as the theory of *yin* and *yang* (*am/duong* in Vietnamese, *um/yang* in Korean, and so on). *Yin*, which represents the negative, dark, cold, feminine side of all things, and *yang*, which represents the positive, bright, warm, masculine side of all things, must remain in balance and harmony. When they are out of harmony, disease and catastrophe occur.

This theory of *yin* and *yang* permeates almost every aspect of the Asian world view, including lifestyle, values, health, and illness. According to this theory, every facet of life and nature is made up of opposite but complementary forces that do not exist apart from one another. Since everything that is *yin* has a small amount of *yang* in it, and vice versa, Asians tend to view things in shades of gray rather than as absolutes. Sometimes this makes it difficult for Asians to accept a Western diagnosis of a single "cause" of a complaint or to rely on a single form of medical treatment or cure.

Confucianism. Confucianism (and neo-Confucianism) concentrates on interpersonal rules and the proper way to conduct social interactions. It reminds people to practice moderation and avoid excess, and to understand that they are destined to fulfill their mission on earth and need to allow *ming*, or fate, to guide their lives.

Reciprocity and loyalty. The key teachings on social interaction are reciprocity, or *pao* (one should treat others as one wants to be treated), and loyalty, or *chung*. These two teachings have led to a respect for authority and a demand for filial piety that manifests itself in most Asian groups by two expectations: that young people will respect and obey the wishes of their parents and other elders, and that one owes unquestioning allegiance and subordination to one's elders and authority figures. Other teachings include benevolence, which involves helping others, and righteousness, which dictates doing what is appropriate and expected.

Gift giving. Western physicians and other caregivers are often taken aback when Asian patients present them with a gift. This custom, too, can be traced to the teachings of Confucius. One expresses good wishes by giving gifts on social occasions and holidays, and an expensive gift enhances one's "face" or shows off one's wealth. Further, it is expected that a gift or favor will be returned; in the physician/patient relationship, the return usually hoped for is good care.

Taboo against the removal of body parts. Another Confucian belief—one that can have a profound effect on an Asian patient's attitude toward surgery—is that "only those shall be truly revered who, at the end of their lives, will return their physical bodies whole and sound." In other words, the body is regarded as being lent to a person during life on earth. Only those who return the body whole at death can expect to go to heaven. Therefore, Asians are not likely to agree easily to removal of any body part or to organ donation.

Buddhism. Buddhism, brought to China from India between 563 and 483 B.C.E., has also shaped the world view and values of most Asians. Out of Buddhist teachings come many attitudes toward life and behavioral traits that may manifest themselves during physician/patient interactions. These include acceptance of fate and suffering, stoicism, behavioral reserve, and suppression of negative thoughts and complaints. Zen Buddhism, which came to Japan from China in the thirteenth century, stresses meditation and enlightenment, which result from intuitive thought, self-discipline, and a direct style of life.

Taoism. Taoism is based upon the philosophy and teachings of Lao Tzu (sometimes translated as "Laotse"), who was born in China about 604 B.C.E. Much of the Asian perspective on health comes from Taoist thought. The central belief of Taoism involves finding the "way," or *tao*. This is achieved by "flowing in accordance with nature" and remaining in harmony with both the cosmological (*yin/yang*) and natural spheres. Following the natural ebb and flow of the universe means that one adopts the *chung-yung*, or golden mean, by maintaining a middle position that avoids extremes.

In many ways, this philosophy advocates noninterference and inaction: learning to detach oneself from the world and allowing things to become what they will. Further, the Taoist cyclical view of nature implies that one should remain in harmony with the changing of the seasons, the waxing and waning of the moon, and the rhythm of night and day. Taoism teaches that life, too, is a cycle consisting of birth, death, and reincarnation; that all things in nature ebb and flow, reaching one extreme (e.g., fortune) and then reverting to the other (e.g., misfortune). The reserve that Asians instinctively show in times of prosperity and the stoicism they display in the face of illness and adversity can be misunderstood by Westerners; caregivers should make every effort to understand and respect these beliefs and attitudes.

HMONG

Hmong Names and Family Ties

There are 18 clan names among the Hmong. All Hmong with the same last name are related. Incest taboos regarding marriage exist for people having the same last name. Men turn to their extended families for assistance in social, political, financial, and health related problems. Men of the same family have greater responsibility to one another than they have to their wives and there is an elaborate system of forms of address that indicates family relationships. Most Hmong men have three names: the clan name (which is placed first in Laos, but is reversed after coming to the United States to follow the Western custom of placing the family name last); the name given to the three-day-old child at the naming ceremony; and an adult name given at a *tis npe laus* ritual that celebrates the rite of passage into manhood. Most women do not receive an adult name. When married, the woman retains her father's clan name and does not adopt her husband's clan name even though she leaves her family and becomes a member of her husband's family.

Health Status

Many Hmong refugees suffer from depression, post-traumatic stress disorder, and culture shock due to their experiences in Laos and Thailand. Many have not been able to adjust to the change from their small self-sufficient agricultural villages to urban life. Many had never seen flush toilets, electricity, or motorized vehicles before their arrival in the United States. Although child mortality has declined, the health status of Hmong adults is deteriorating. The health of Hmong adults in California is reported to be worse than that of comparable Hmong living in primitive conditions in Thailand. There is a twofold increase in the number of respiratory complaints, twenty times the incidence of diabetes and hypertension, and thirteen times the incidence of mental distress and depression. Seventy-nine percent of adult Hmong living in Fresno, California, are overweight. This deterioration in health may be partially attributed to changes in lifestyle and eating habits and to the inability to adjust to a breakdown in the traditional social system. The matrilineal, patrilocal, and patriarchal society, as well as their way of life, has been destroyed. Elders have to rely on children's knowledge of English and American ways and are no longer respected for their wisdom.

Traditional healing methods such as coining, cupping, massage, soul calling, ritual healing, and use of herbal therapies are still frequently used by Hmong living in the United States. Family members may bring traditional medicines and ritual healing to a hospital bedside. Some Christian Hmong may substitute Christian prayer groups for the traditional shaman. Whenever traditional prayer and/or Western medicine fails to result in a cure, the family often turn to animistic cures.

Traditional Beliefs about Body Functions

Each body part is essential to the whole of the body and, as such, each has a soul. Because the brain is the thinking center and protects the body, the anterior fontanel is considered sacred and may not be washed until it hardens. The Hmong, along with other Asian groups, consider the head to be sacred. Casual touching of a person's head by others, such as an adult rubbing a child's head, is considered disrespectful and degrading. The soul, which is reincarnated, lies in the heart, which provides the body with blood and life. However, unlike in Western culture, the liver, not the heart, is the seat of emotions. One half of the liver represents goodness and the other badness. When the larger half of the liver represents goodness, the person is good-hearted, and vice versa. Hmong share the traditional Chinese belief that blood is finite and not replenished. Hmong, therefore, may oppose blood draws because they believe that loss of too much blood will make a person weak.

It is important to note that certain Hmong phrases denoting parts of the body do not directly correspond to the names used in English. Medical oversights and errors can be avoided by making sure that a professionally trained interpreter is present during examinations.

Spiritual and Non-Spiritual Causes of Disease in Hmong Culture

A study of the beliefs of Hmong mothers regarding the causes of disease states that they consider environmental elements and unsuitable food or drink to be non-spiritual causes of illness and "soul loss" to be a spiritual cause of illness.

When illness is believed to have been caused by spirits, it will be treated by traditional cures such as soul calling and ancestral worship. Measles, an important health problem for Hmong children, is believed to be related to seasonal weather cycles and brought on strong wind. When a child has measles, a faith healer called a *khawv koob* may be called in to conduct a ritual called *ua neeb*. This ritual is intended to open communication with the spirit causing the measles. The healer asks the spirit to come out of the child's body. If the child shows a rash during the next three-day period, the child is taken to a physician. Strong-smelling foods, such as fried foods, are not prepared when the household has a child suffering from measles, and an effort is made to retain the child's body heat.

Non-spiritually caused illnesses are treated both by over-the-counter Western medicines (one such popular medicine is Pepto Bismol) and by herbs and plants such as dry wood, plant roots, sida leaf, and tea. Animal-based remedies, such as dried rhinoceros horn and cow gallbladder, are also used in water to prepare a medicinal drink. Sometimes rhinoceros feces (available at ethnic retail stores) are rubbed on the child's abdomen or a shaman is asked to concoct a special remedy. A mother may also decrease the amount of milk given to a child suffering from diarrhea.

SOUTH ASIANS: INDIA, PAKISTAN, BANGLADESH, AND SRI LANKA

South Asians are extremely diverse, especially in regard to religion, culture, and language. The primary religious/cultural groups are Hindus, Sikhs, and Muslims. Although many people from these cultural groups will require interpreters who speak their local dialect, many will list English as their first or primary language. Being a native English speaker does not preclude communication barriers. Many English-speaking South Asians will be unfamiliar with many American words, expressions, and idioms. Care needs to be taken to avoid idiomatic expressions and ensure that information and instructions have been correctly understood. Because education is more highly stressed for males than females, women may be less fluent in English than men. If an interpreter is needed, it is advisable to obtain someone of the same gender and at least as old as the patient.

India was the second most frequent country of origin for immigrants to the United States from 2001 to 2003. A very large majority of Indian immigrants (83.8 percent) have a minimum of a high school diploma. A husband will often try to show caring for the welfare of his wife by speaking for her even if she is fluent in English. Modesty, humility, shyness, tolerance, and silence are emphasized from early childhood and affection and caring are expressed through the eyes and facial expressions rather than through touching. Direct eye contact may be avoided, especially by the elderly, because it can be viewed as rude or a sign of disrespect. Men are generally more familiar and comfortable with shaking hands than women.

Sikhism has one of the largest religious followings in India. Like Indians of other faiths, Sikhs have immigrated to the United States and have continued to follow their religious beliefs. The Sikh religion forbids Sikh males to cut or shave any body hair; thus, in spite of the Western medical custom of shaving a surgical area prior to surgery to reduce the possibility of infection, whenever possible the area should be cleansed without removing any body hair. In cases where removal is absolutely necessary, this must be carefully explained to both the patient and his or her family and permission should be obtained beforehand. Sikh men wear a *kirpan* (a piece of cloth worn on the chest), a *kanga* (a wooden comb), and a *kara* (an iron bracelet). For Sikhs and other religious groups, such as Hindus and Muslims, items worn for religious purposes should never be removed without first obtaining permission.

Most South Asians are used to a peri-wash with water after elimination and Muslims must use their left hand to wipe this area (as the right hand is used for eating). Strict Muslims must wash to purify themselves prior to prayer. Traditionally Hindus are vegetarian. Some may fast one day a week or month to purify themselves. Muslims fast from sunrise to sunset during the month of Ramadan.

"Hot"/"Cold" Beliefs

Those who believe in Ayurvedic medicine share similar beliefs in the "hot" and "cold" classification system as described above in the section on traditional Chinese health beliefs. "Hot" spices include pepper, clove, cinnamon, mustard, garlic, and ginger, while "cold" spices include cardamom and fennel seed. Mango and papaya are "hot" fruits, while lemons, oranges, bananas, and tomatoes are "cold" fruits. Among dairy products, cheese and eggs are considered "hot" and yogurt and ice cream are considered "cold." Pregnancy is considered a "hot" state so "cooling" foods such as milk products and "cold" fruits and vegetables are encouraged. "Hot" foods such as pepper and papaya are to be avoided by pregnant women because they are thought to induce premature labor. It is recommended that "cold" foods such as yogurt and banana not be eaten at night because they are believed to cause a cold or a sore throat. It should be noted that in some cases these beliefs are supported by Western medical knowledge. For example, papaya does contain an alkaloid that can stimulate uterine contractions and bananas can trigger an asthmatic attack in those prone to asthma.

Sexuality, Fertility, and Childbirth

Male as well as female patients from this region may not have had any formal sex education and may be lacking in even the basic knowledge of human reproduction commonly assumed by caregivers in the U.S. healthcare system. Emphasis on the person's role in and duty to society, the custom of prearranged marriage, and the importance of the family and the birth of the first child may have left issues such as conception and contraceptive education to chance. One study (see Fisher et al.) even reports a case of a couple seeking assistance for infertility after an eleven-year marriage that had not been consummated. Neither the man nor the woman had thought to inform the physician of that fact and it was only discovered after the woman was convinced to undergo a pelvic examination. The couple were highly educated and the husband held a doctoral degree. This story illustrates that what may be assumed to be common knowledge in one culture is not necessarily so in another. Caregivers need to check patients' knowledge rather than draw assumptions based upon their own cultural backgrounds.

FILIPINOS

According to the 2000 census there are 1,850,314 Filipinos living in the United States. The word "Filipino" is an anglicized form of "Pilipino" as there is no "f" in the Pilipino language. For all practical purposes, there are eight major languages of Malayo-Indonesian origin, though as many as 87 dialects have been identified. The official language is Pilipino, which is based upon Tagalog with Malayo-Indonesian, Chinese, Spanish, and English words intermingled. From 1898 until recently, English was the language of instruction in the schools, and it is now widely taught as a second language. Though English is spoken by the majority of Filipinos living in the United States, most speak it with a heavy accent and are very affected by the tone and manner of the person speaking to them.

The Philippines is an island country comprised of approximately 7,000 islands that are geographically part of Asia. The first settlers are believed to have been Negritos. Indo-Malayans began arriving about 4000 B.C.E. and continued arriving until the fourteenth century C.E., when Japanese and Chinese traders began to arrive. In 1521 Ferdinand Magellan arrived, naming the islands the Philippines after Philip II of Spain. The Philippines remained a Spanish possession until after the Spanish-American War of 1898, and did not become a free republic until July 4, 1946. This influx of cultures and mixture of conquerors has resulted in the development of a very unique culture.

Filipinos (or Philipinos) tend to be shy and affectionate, very soft-spoken, and not given to voicing disagreement. The culture advocates respect and obedience toward parents and authority figures (such as physicians and nurses); direct eye contact with authority figures is avoided. A polite request is more common than a command. The family is very important and a close family member should be consulted before a negative prognosis is given to the patient. Filipino self-esteem is dependent upon fulfilling obligations to and gaining the approval of family. Rural farming villages or barrios were the major form of social structure in all but big cities such as Manila. This has influenced the development of cultural values such as family, neighborliness, and community solidarity. For example, even today in Filipino communities in Hawaii (where the greatest number of Filipinos reside outside the Philippines itself), a baby may have as many as 30 godparents. The majority of Filipinos are Roman Catholics (although there are some Protestants and Muslims) and religion usually plays an important role in Filipino life. Often, when a person becomes ill, a priest as well as a physician is called.

Illness Beliefs

Although literature pertaining to Filipino health beliefs does not refer to either *yin/yang* or "hot"/"cold" dichotomies, illness is generally believed to be caused by an imbalance of spirit or moral elements (bad behavior or punishment). Filipinos tend to ignore illness until it is quite advanced or pain becomes unbearable. For many, illness and suffering are regarded as unavoidable conditions of life. When ill, the Filipino patient tends to assume a passive role and expects decisions to be made for him or her. Chinese influence on Filipino culture makes it common for many to try herbal remedies prior to consulting a physician, but once a physician is consulted, there tends to be great respect for and compliance with the Western medical approach. Good health is related to balance, and good eating (not necessarily healthful eating) is important to health. Being overweight is often seen as proof of high socioeconomic standing and exercise is not a tradition in Filipino culture.

DEVELOPING CULTURAL PERSPECTIVE

1. Why might the family of a hospitalized Asian patient ask if they can bring meals to the patient?

2. By law, caregivers are mandated reporters and must report any signs of suspected abuse. The results of several traditional Asian medical treatments might lead the caregiver to suspect abuse. What are these treatments and why would abuse be suspected?

3. Why would an Asian patient be unlikely to sign an organ donor card?

4. List ways to ensure that an Asian patient understands the importance of his/her independent treatment regimen.

5. Why would a patient who is a traditional Hmong resist giving multiple samples of blood?

6. What would be the most culturally acceptable way to inform a Filipino patient of a negative prognosis or a treatment regimen?

BLENDING PERSPECTIVES

1. Refer to Review question 2 on mandated reporting. Do existing policies need to be modified to accommodate different treatment systems? Why or why not?

2. Considering the theory of *yin* and *yang*, is Western medicine too simplistic in assigning a "cause" to a particular disease?

3. How does the theory of *yin* and *yang* relate to traditional Asian concepts of "hot" and "cold"? How does this relate to "the golden mean" or moderation in all things?

Chapter

5

Providing Culture-Sensitive Healthcare to Hispanic/Latino Patients

On the use of the term Hispanic *versus* Latino: The term *Hispanic* has been used in this guide because it is generally more familiar to providers than the term *Latino*. However, it is important to understand that the term *Hispanic* is an artificial designation that was created by the U.S. Census Bureau in 1970 as an ethnic category for persons who identify themselves as being of Spanish origin. The term *Latino* first appeared in the U.S. Census in 2000, when all respondents were asked to identify whether their ethnicity was of *Spanish/Hispanic/Latino* origin. The term *Latino* is the one that most people of Latin American origin use to refer to themselves. It is also important to recognize that both terms refer to an extremely diverse group. While the majority is of Mexican origin (58 percent according to the 2000 Census), the group referred to as *Hispanic* or *Latino* also includes persons of Puerto Rican, Cuban, Central American, Dominican, or other Hispanic origin. Furthermore, while all may be united by the Spanish language (except those of Brazilian origin, who speak Portuguese), the language is spoken with a great variation in dialects, accents, and syntax. These variations may affect communication between Spanish speakers regarding parts of the body, bodily functions, symptoms of illness, and health practices. As is the case with all the other population groups discussed in this book, it is important to refrain from making assumptions regarding the cultural and healthcare beliefs and practices of individual patients based primarily on the fact that they may have a Hispanic family name. The degree of adherence to Hispanic culture or assimilation to mainstream U.S. culture should be carefully assessed for each individual patient.

Keys to a Good Professional Relationship with Hispanic Patients

1. *Show* respeto. People from many Hispanic cultures offer (and expect to receive) deference on the basis of age, sex, and status. Patients will naturally offer *respeto* to the health provider, an authority figure with high social, educational, and economic status. In return, patients rightfully expect to be treated

with respect as defined by Hispanic rules of etiquette.

The health provider shows *respeto* by:

- addressing adults by title and family name (Mr./*Señor* X, Mrs./*Señora* Y, or Madam/*Doña*).
- shaking hands at the beginning of each meeting.
- using *usted* rather than the informal *tu* for "you," if addressing them in Spanish.
- making eye contact, without necessarily expecting reciprocation, since some (especially rural) patients may consider it disrespectful to look the health provider, an authority figure, in the eye.
- speaking directly to the patient, even when speaking through an interpreter.
- refraining from smiling or showing any disbelief or ridicule while the patient is attempting to describe a health belief (such as the cause of an illness) or an alternative (folk) form of cure.

2. *Be* simpatico. *Simpatia* is the Spanish word for kindness. It is shown by politeness and "pleasantness in the face."

The health provider shows *simpatia* by:

- engaging the patient and showing a genuine interest in him or her, as a neutral or detached attitude may be interpreted as a lack of caring, and this may make the patient loath to share details of his or her complaint.
- emphasizing courtesy and following social amenities, such as shaking hands, touching (a pat on the back, a tap on the shoulder, etc.), and asking about the patient's personal life.

3. *Show* personalismo. Patients from most Hispanic cultures will respond more positively to caregivers if a one-on-one relationship is established. This is not to be confused with an informal relationship, i.e., one that is anything less than fully professional. Although establishing a relationship based on *personalismo* may seem time-consuming, it can actually save time and prevent negative outcomes that can result from misunderstanding of treatment or noncompliance with care.

The health provider shows *personalismo* by:

- treating patients in a warm and friendly—but not in an unduly informal—manner.
- showing genuine interest in and concern for patients by asking them about themselves and their family.
- sitting close, leaning forward, and using gestures when speaking with patients.

4. *Involve the family in decision making and care. Familism* represents a major value of Hispanics, who view family obligations as primary. The family provides and helps in the form of material and emotional support. Family members are expected to assist in solving problems and in making all important decisions.

Note that the definition of *la familia* is much broader in most Hispanic cultures than in Anglo cultures and may include not only parents and siblings, but also grandparents, cousins, aunts and uncles, and even close family friends.

La familia may demonstrate their loyalty and support by gathering at the hospital. Health providers should understand that there may be noise and confusion (by U.S. standards) that results from "the gathering of the clan." Try to accommodate their presence without impinging on the care of other patients, since they contribute a great deal to both the patient's and the family's sense of well-being.

5. *Accept a different sense of time.* Many people from Hispanic cultures have what might be called a "global" or "indefinite" sense of time—rather than an

exact sense of day and hour—in making and keeping appointments. Similarly, in presenting a complaint, they may not be able to attach a specific calendar date to the onset or conclusion of a medical complaint or an event such as menses or conception. They may instead be able to link the event to a season, a phase of the moon, or a particular occurrence, such as a holiday or celebration.

6. *Take pains to establish understanding and agreement.* Many patients' sense of respect for authority may cause them to avoid conflict or confrontation with the health provider by saying too readily that they understand how to take a medication or will follow a treatment plan. The health provider must ensure that understanding is achieved and must try to gain real acceptance of the treatment plan and a commitment to follow it.

7. *Respect the spiritual side of physical complaints.* Many Hispanic patients complain that health practitioners, by discounting supernatural and psychological causes of complaints, offer only a fragmentary approach to care. To these patients, this amounts to treating the symptoms, not the disease itself. Practitioners are advised to ask their patients what *they* believe to be the cause of a complaint and to refrain from ridiculing or discounting the patient's belief in supernatural or psychological causes.

8. *Accept fatalism.* This is a common Hispanic belief that the individual can do little to alter fate. Work with this notion by suggesting:
   - ways that the patient may assist God in keeping him or her well; and
   - how taking care of oneself helps the person to be there to support his or her family.

Health Problems and Concerns Common to Members of Hispanic Culture

Persons from some Hispanic cultures may have a tendency toward certain health concerns due to cultural factors, as listed below. Many of these concerns are derived from the chapter entitled "Latino Health Status" by Olivia Carter-Pokras and Ruth Enid Zambrana in *Health Issues in the Latino Community*.

Specific concerns include:

1. *a high incidence of teenage pregnancy* among Mexican and Puerto Rican populations. According to data published in 2000 by the National Center for Health Statistics, the percentage of Mexican and Puerto Rican teenagers under the age of 18 who become pregnant is twice that of Whites;

2. *a low incidence of breast-feeding,* especially in the Puerto Rican population;

3. *where breast-feeding is practiced, a tendency to do so for a short period* and to introduce solid foods earlier than recommended in current pediatric guidelines;

4. *a very low intake of vitamin A;*

5. *alcohol abuse,* especially by young Hispanic males (abetted by cultural taboos against female disclosure of alcohol use);

6. *drug use* at levels higher than among non-Hispanic Whites;

7. *a high prevalence of undetected non-insulin-dependent diabetes* (especially among Mexicans with Pima Indian blood);

8. *a high incidence of tuberculosis* (the National Alliance for Hispanic Health [NAHH]—formerly the National Coalition of Hispanic Health and Human Services Organizations, or COSSMHO—recommends aggressive screening with the Mantoux tuberculin skin test and, if the test is positive, use of the National Institutes of Health's [NIH] preventive therapy, because of the high use of the bacille Calmette-Guérin [BCG] antituberculosis vaccine in Latin America);

9. *a high risk for mental health problems* such as depression, anxiety, and substance abuse;

10. *dietary concerns* due to:
    - a high consumption of fats (often lard, especially for low-income people) and fried food;
    - a traditional diet high in carbohydrates from beans and rice (Puerto Rico, Cuba, and the Caribbean islands) or corn tortilla (Mexico); and
    - low intake of green or leafy vegetables and/or milk and eggs, especially in conjunction with increased consumption of meat and fast foods as acculturation occurs;
11. *lack of sunshine* (primarily for immigrants to northern cities);
12. *little tradition for "recreational" physical exercise* outside the context of field or other physical labor;
13. *excessive reliance on Azarcon* (also called "Greta" or "Alarcon"), which is about 90 percent lead, as a home remedy for gastrointestinal/intestinal complaints; and
14. *sharing of hypodermic needles and syringes* with family and friends, which in Mexico are often used to administer vitamins, medications, and contraceptives.

Folk Beliefs about Health and Illness That Can Affect Care and Treatment

1. *Good health is a matter of luck that can easily change.* Sick persons may be the innocent victims of "fate," with little responsibility for taking action to regain health.
2. *Negative forces and punishment.* Illness may be the result of negative forces in the environment or a punishment for transgressions.
3. *Balance and harmony are important to health and well-being.* Illness may be the result of an imbalance.
4. *The natural and supernatural worlds are not clearly distinguishable, and body and soul are inseparable.* Telling a patient that an illness is all in the mind is meaningless because there is little or no distinction between somatic and psychosomatic illness.
5. *Cure requires family participation and support.* The family's role is to indulge the patient, provide unconditional love and support, and participate in health-care decision making.
6. *Caregiver's gift or calling.* While education and training may be somewhat important, what truly matters is the caregiver's "gift" or "calling" for curing illness.
7. *Healing effects of demonstrating pain.* Moaning, far from being a sign of low tolerance to pain, is a culturally accepted way to reduce pain and to share it with interested others.
8. *Classification of diseases.* Diseases may be divided into Anglo and traditional diseases, and traditional diseases may be either natural or unnatural. Many people mix and match "modern" medicine and traditional care, consulting modern health providers for Anglo and natural diseases, and folk healers for unnatural diseases.

Major Folk Illnesses among Hispanic Populations

Ataque. A culturally condoned emotional response to a great shock or bad news, characterized by hyperventilation, bizarre behavior, violence, and/or an inability to speak.

Bilis. An illness believed to be caused by strong emotions that result in an imbalance of bile, which "boils over" into the bloodstream. Symptoms include vomiting, diarrhea, headaches, dizziness, and/or migraine headaches.

Diseases of "hot"/"cold" imbalance. The "hot"/"cold" theory of disease traces its roots to the Aristotelian system of humors, which were either "hot" or "cold," "wet" or "dry." The "hot"/"cold" portion of the theory survives in many Hispanics of Mexican and Puerto Rican origin. Body organs, diseases, foods, and liquids may be "hot" or "cold," and good health depends on maintaining a balance of "hot" and "cold." A "hot" ailment calls for "cold" herbs and foods to restore the balance, and vice versa.

It is important to note that temperature is not the key factor in the classification scheme. Ice is "hot" because it can burn, and Linden tea, though served hot, is "cold" and is often used by Mexicans to treat "hot" ailments. Penicillin, neutral in temperature, is considered "hot" because it may cause "hot" symptoms, such as diarrhea or rash.

Acceptance of the "hot"/"cold" system can affect compliance with treatment. For instance, a patient suffering from a high fever may resist cold compresses, reacting against the treatment of a "hot" ailment (fever) with a "hot" treatment (ice).

Indirect questions can help a provider determine whether a patient subscribes to the "hot"/"cold" belief system. If the patient does, the provider is advised to try to work within the "hot"/"cold" framework to increase patient trust and maximize compliance.

Mollera cerrado or *cerrado de mollera* (fallen fontanel). A condition believed to exist when an infant's anterior fontanel is either visibly depressed or believed to have been depressed as the result of trauma. Symptoms are excessive crying, lack of desire or ability to feed, diarrhea, vomiting, restlessness, and irritability. Whether real or imagined, this problem warrants attention because the family may believe it to be fatal if not treated.

Mal de ojo (evil eye). A spell usually cast on a child when a person with the evil eye admires the child without touching it. Children are often protected by special earrings, necklaces, amulets, or other jewelry, which should not be removed from the child's person during examinations. The most common treatment is prayer while sweeping the child's body with a mixture of eggs, lemons, and bay leaves— a treatment called *limpia* in Mexico and *barrida* in Puerto Rico. This process is also used to diagnose *mal de ojo*.

Susto (soul loss). A disease that can attack anyone, regardless of gender, age, racial group, or economic status, believed to result from a series of overwhelming events that causes the soul to become dislodged and escape from the body. It is manifested by a number of clinically diagnosed diseases, including cancer, kidney failure, diabetes, and high blood pressure. The variety of symptoms and pathologies through which *susto* is manifested absolves patients and relatives of any "guilt" for failing to take timely precautions or seek treatment for the disease. A long time is usually said to elapse between the event or events and the physical manifestations of *susto*. Many Hispanics of both rural and urban backgrounds accept this theory, regardless of how it is manifested.

Embrujado (roughly translated as "bewitchment"). A socially accepted psychological disease (in contrast to being considered "mad"), *embrujado* may be manifested through physical or psychological illness, depending on the intent of the bewitcher (who is always female). Some researchers have suggested that *embrujado* may be a culturally accepted behavior for males who cannot cope with the Anglo world.

Major Systems of Folk Healing among Hispanic Populations

Curanderismo. A system of care derived from a mixture of Aztec, Spanish, spiritualistic, homeopathic, and modern medicine, *curanderismo* is used to treat physical, psychological, and social illnesses. Used throughout Latin America, it is more widely practiced by Mexican immigrants than by Puerto Rican, Cuban, and Caribbean immigrant groups. There is also considerable diversity in *curanderismo* according to regional culture.

Curanderismo shares many scientific concepts and procedures with modern scientific medicine, and health practitioners should beware of dismissing it as "quackery." In fact, because of the major role *curanderismo* plays in Hispanic health beliefs and practices, hospitals and clinics in metropolitan areas with large Hispanic populations are beginning to cooperate with *curanderos*—sometimes even placing them on hospital staff.

A practitioner is either a *curandero* (male) or a *curandera* (female), and may be a member of the patient's nuclear or extended family. Sometimes the *curandera* is a *señora* or older woman who has developed a reputation for success in treating friends and family. Sometimes the *curandero* is a *sobador,* a male who heals through massage (although this is less frequent in the United States than in Mexico). A *partera*, or midwife, is often used in Mexico (and less often by Mexican immigrants in the United States) because a woman is believed to have a better understanding of the female reproductive system than any man, including a "scientific" physician.

Santero or *brujería.* A structured system of healing magic that originated in what is now Nigeria. When brought to Puerto Rico, Cuba, and Brazil by African slaves, who were later converted to Catholicism, *santero* became fused with the Catholic system of saints and imagery.

The *santero,* a religious healer or "spiritualist," performs religious or magical ceremonies, administers potions, and prepares amulets. In Spanish Harlem in New York, parts of Florida, and others areas heavily populated by Puerto Ricans, Cubans, or people from the Caribbean, *santeros* often practice *espiritismo* in storefronts, basements, homes, and similar locations. People can also purchase herbs, potions, and charms at a *botanica* without consulting a healer.

Estimates vary as to the extent to which folk healers and cures are used by Hispanics in the United States, ranging from a low estimate of 4 percent nationwide to a high of 73 percent in a survey of mental health patients at a Los Angeles clinic. As a general rule, providers may assume that Hispanic patients who come to them after having delayed seeking healthcare for an inordinate length of time may have unsuccessfully tried a folk healing system first. On the other hand, patients who disappear after receiving a negative prognosis or failing to experience an immediate cure may have left the healthcare system for some form of folk healing. Often, however, they return so late that successful treatment is no longer possible.

DEVELOPING CULTURAL PERSPECTIVE

1. What cultural traditions would influence the response to the advice, "get more exercise"?

2. Why would a Hispanic patient with a high fever resist a cold compress?

3. Why would a depressed anterior fontanel on an infant cause alarm to the family?

4. Explain why the concept of *susto* (soul loss) might cause a patient to delay seeking treatment for a serious illness.

BLENDING PERSPECTIVES

1. How do you view illness? Is it a matter of genetics? Environment? Luck? Diet? How does the Hispanic view differ from yours?

2. Are you comfortable with the Hispanic belief in "evil influences"? Do you feel comfortable speaking with a patient about this subject? Do you think talking about "evil" conflicts with the general prohibition against mixing religion with medicine?

6

Providing Culture-Sensitive Healthcare to People from the Middle East

Over the past twenty years, significant numbers of people from the Middle East have immigrated to the United States. While not all of these people are Arabs (such as Iranians, who are Persians), most are Muslims. The U.S. Muslim population is estimated to be 3 to 4 million, with most of this population coming from Pakistan, Iran, Iraq, and Indonesia.

Keys to Establishing Successful Relationships with Middle Eastern Patients

1. *Greet patient and family members by title and say something personal about the patient, the patient's family, or the patient's country of origin.* Muslims may not feel comfortable shaking hands, especially with members of the opposite sex. A gesture of acknowledgement rather than a handshake may make the patient feel more at ease. (Reminder: There is great diversity within the groups referred to as "Middle Eastern" and pride attached to region of origin.)

2. *Personalize your relationship with the patient.* Affiliation is a key social need. Because trust is closely tied to the caring involvement of one's "inner circle" of friends and extended family, those defined as strangers or "outsiders" are often viewed with mistrust. Modesty and lack of trust can affect patient care by inhibiting the patient from disclosing information to a caregiver.

3. *Share some information about yourself with the patient.* Sharing such information will help to build trust.

4. *If you feel the patient may be withholding information, use indirect questioning to obtain the information you need.* Many patients from the Middle East have great respect for Western medicine and may expect you to "know" information about the patient that the patient has not explicitly told you. Middle Eastern culture is what is known as a "high-context culture"—one in which people are assumed to deduce meaning and information from the context of the situation.

5. *If it's necessary to use an interpreter, use someone who is of the same sex as the patient.* Although it is *never advisable* to use a family member to interpret,

if a family member is asked to interpret because no professional is available, be aware that he or she may "edit" what is being said in order to protect the patient from bad news.

6. *Take the history and physical in stages during, rather than prior to, your examination.* Many patients from the Middle East may resent the detailed questions asked during the standard history and physical because they cannot see their direct relationship with the current complaint. One barrier to patient disclosure of information is a reluctance to disclose personal information to strangers; another is that the high respect for Western medicine may lead some patients to wonder why the physician can't diagnose the illness without "irrelevant" tests and questions.

7. *Do not interpret the loud voice of a patient or family member as anger or displeasure with treatment.* Speaking loudly is a means of demonstrating the importance of the matter, not a reflection of anger (which is traditionally expressed by a high-pitched, intense voice).

8. *Include the family, especially older male relatives, in the medical decision-making process.* Autonomous decision-making is not part of most Middle Eastern cultures. The major responsibility for decisions in many Middle Eastern families rests with the family, for whom the father or the oldest male is expected to act as the spokesperson.

9. *Double-check the patient's intention to follow instructions.* Many patients from the Middle East may seem passive and will probably not question treatment decisions. This is because the physician (especially an older male physician) is viewed as an authority figure who should not be questioned or contradicted. This failure to challenge the physician does not necessarily mean that the patient has accepted a diagnosis and will comply with medical advice.

10. *Don't be put off if the patient or the patient's family members seem to move closer to you and invade your sense of personal space.* For many people from the Middle East, the physical "comfort zone" for any sort of personal interaction is much closer than that of most other groups—especially Americans. "Nose to nose" contact during conversation is not meant aggressively or as a personal offense. It's best to "grin and bear" this contact or place yourself behind a desk or other object so the patient cannot physically move closer to you.

Establishing Trust

Of key importance to most people from the Middle East is the need for affiliation and close ties with family members. The patient's extensive set of relationships with family and friends provides the first source of support and advice during any illness or health crisis. Anyone outside this "inner circle," including health professionals, is often viewed with lack of trust. However, it is fairly easy for a caregiver to move from the position of stranger to trusted affiliate. Once this trust is established, the patient and family may have expectations that will seem "out of bounds" to most Western caregivers.

Trust is usually established only when a personal relationship between the caregiver and the patient and his or her family is formed. Because people are measured not so much as individuals, but as members of families, groups, professional organizations, and even universities, it is important for the Middle Eastern patient to be able to "place" the caregiver in one or more respected groups for trust to develop. A caregiver who takes the time to "warm up" the patient by exchanging a few questions about his or her personal life and family, and disclose something personal, will develop a positive relationship much sooner than one who limits discussion to the specific and formal purpose of the visit.

The sharing of food and drink are also an important means of establishing relationships. The caregiver who offers the Middle Eastern patient a cup of tea during the visit or who accepts a patient's gift of a Middle Eastern sweet will establish a positive beginning. *Note*: If offered a cup of tea, the patient is likely to refuse the first offer. This is because it is considered impolite to accept the initial offer of food or drink. It is important, therefore, to repeat the offer a second or even a third time.

The development of the type of personal relationship important to successful interaction with a Middle Eastern patient is time-consuming. An appointment with a Middle Eastern patient will take longer than that of most other patients, so appointment schedules should be arranged accordingly.

The Role of the Family

The immediate and extended family forms the most important social institution in the Middle East. Parents are expected to care for children until they are married. Children are expected to remain in close contact with their parents after marriage and to care for them in their old age. The family structure is patriarchal. Even adult children are expected to submit to the father's authority. The family institution is maintained with daily contact through spontaneous visits and gatherings.

This close family structure often breaks down when people from the Middle East immigrate to the United States. Family members often live far from one another. In addition, the normal size of apartments or homes makes multigenerational living arrangements very difficult. As a result, children become more independent and aging parents often experience a strong feeling of isolation and abandonment.

In some countries (such as Kuwait and Saudi Arabia), men tend to gather with other men in cafes, while women gather in the home. In more liberated countries such as Egypt, gatherings are not segregated by gender. These gatherings are not only social. They serve many important functions—one of which is to provide support during times of illness. Members can turn to others without formally requesting help. It is customary to share problems in the course of general conversation. Advice and help are expected and given without any specific request.

Offering and Taking Medical Advice

Caregivers in the Middle East typically assess and analyze the patient's medical condition and needs but, instead of offering specific advice, suggest a number of treatment options from which the patient is asked to choose. When these choices are given to the unassimilated Middle Eastern patient, they often will be rejected. Like the first offer of tea or refreshment, this rejection is not meant as a refusal of care. The caregiver should repeat the offer with greater insistence. The patient may either accept one of the choices or seek help within the system or from other "affiliates" outside of it.

Language and Communication Style

In spite of differences in local dialect, most Arab Americans are able to understand one another (with special exceptions such as Yemenites, who speak a local dialect not readily understood by other Arabs). One source likens the difference between Egyptian Arabic and non-Egyptian Arabic to the difference between American and British English—these groups are able to understand one another in spite of differences in language style and common expressions. Although the written languages of Arabs and Iranians are very similar, these groups are not able to understand each other's spoken language.

Warmth with Intimates versus Courtesy with Outsiders

Although people from the Middle East tend to be warm and expressive toward intimates, they treat strangers with a ritual courtesy that is often misunderstood as friendship by outsiders. The statement, "My house is your house" is only a formula. It is used with strangers but not with intimates. On the other hand, close family and friends know, without having to be told, that material goods are common property within a person's inner circle of intimates. A Middle Easterner would risk his or her life to help another member of this inner circle.

Masking One's Own Motives and Reading the Motives of Others

Within the Middle Eastern cultures discussed in this chapter, there is a stress on appearing polite and a desire to please others. Iranians value a type of personal cleverness that masks the correct interpretation of their actions by others but allows them to successfully interpret the actions of others.

Knowing and Seeing the "Right" People

Social and professional standing are valued very highly and it is not uncommon for Middle Eastern patients and/or their families to demand to see the "head of the department" or the caregiver reputed to be the "top person in his or her field." The importance given to social status also makes people from the Middle East interested in learning not only, "Who is your family?" but also, "Who do you know of importance?" A little personal information goes a long way in developing a warmer relationship with these patients.

Communicating Medical Problems to Caregivers

Most people from the Middle East are very modest and value privacy. Therefore, they have a strong resistance to disclosing personal information to strangers. They are likely to resent the physician's history and physical or the health assessment upon admission to a hospital as a gross invasion of privacy. Because this hesitancy to disclose information is dispelled as soon as a more personal relationship with the caregiver is established, it is advised that the caregiver wait to solicit information not needed immediately.

Patients are often vague in the information they do provide, not only due to language difficulties, but also because they are unfamiliar with concepts that distinguish mental from physical conditions. They often lack experience in describing symptoms in relation to specific parts of the body.

These difficulties are compounded by a view of the caregiver as an authority figure. The caregiver's views are never outwardly questioned or challenged. The patient tends to remain passive in the physician's presence. This desire to show "proper respect" includes refraining from asking any questions that might challenge the physician's authority as well as the presentation of any information that might contradict a health professional's diagnosis. Respect for health professionals also makes it difficult for many people from the Middle East to understand the need for tests and (what they consider) irrelevant questions. After all, the physician should have the expertise to make a diagnosis without further exploration.

What Is Meant When the Patient Repeats What He Says and Raises His Voice

Members of many Middle Eastern cultures often use repetition as a means of stressing the importance of something that is said in the hope of increasing the listeners' understanding of the message. Although this is often interpreted by

Americans as meaningless redundancy, it is a way of emphasizing the importance of a subject and is a communication pattern that is characteristic of Muslim prayers. Caregivers can reassure patients of their understanding of the message by nodding and repeating that message in their own words. Another way of conveying the importance of what is being said is in the degree of loudness with which one speaks. The louder the voice, the more important the speaker perceives the message to be. Anger, on the other hand, is usually expressed by a high-pitched, intense voice.

Patients from the Middle East and their families are often characterized as "demanding" because of their tendency to speak loudly. This increased volume is used to indicate the importance of what is being said. Demanding behavior by family and friends is prescribed by the culture. It is intended to show their level of caring for the patient. It is also the role of the family to insist upon the best care possible for the family member by constantly engaging the caregiver, remaining by the patient's side at all times, and showering the patient with care and affection.

Interaction and Disclosure in a High-Context Culture

Many people from the Middle East tend to understand events in the context of the situation in which they occur rather than through the verbal message that accompanies or describes the events. The critical importance of context in Middle Eastern culture may lead patients to ignore or to avoid the matter at hand until a better context for sharing is established between caregiver and patient. The caregiver should also keep in mind that in verbal messages, form is of greater importance than the content (the words) of the message. Patients from the Middle East find it easier to share information and feelings with members of the same gender. This is especially true because an important aspect of sharing is through "touch," which is only permitted by members of the same sex.

Body language and eye contact are also important communicators, and health practitioners are advised to pay careful attention to these forms of nonverbal communication when in conference with Middle Eastern patients and/or their families.

Orientations to Time and Space

People from the Middle East tend to be more past- and present-oriented than future-oriented. Although they may arrive on time for official engagements such as appointments with physicians, they are more spontaneous about time in social and informal gatherings.

Planning ahead is an American and Western European value foreign to many people from the Middle East. Planning may be viewed as an effort to defy Allah's will or to bring on the evil eye or other negative conditions. Therefore, it is rare for women from Middle Eastern cultures to buy clothing or fix up a room for an unborn child. A person with a fatal illness will tend to avoid making any sort of preparation for death. Birth control or other types of family planning are also viewed as going against Allah's will and tempting fate.

The conversational space needs of Westerners are much greater than those of many people from the Middle East. The appropriate conversational distance for people from the Middle East is about two feet from the person with whom they are speaking, while for Americans it is about five feet. Caregivers tend to feel uncomfortable and "threatened" when patients seem to move in on them to hold a conversation. This feeling of being threatened or attacked is exacerbated if the patient or the family member raises his or her voice to emphasize the importance of what is being said. These differences in kinetics and appropriate tone of voice often make it difficult for caregivers to avoid developing negative attitudes toward their patients from the Middle East.

Disclosing Medical Information or Bad News to the Patient and Patient's Family

When medical information is communicated to the patient, it is important to include a family head or spokesperson. This spokesperson is usually the oldest male present. If no male is present, the spokesperson may be a female, although females are considered more emotionally susceptible to bad news.

In Middle Eastern cultures, negative information is usually presented in stages. The withholding of a negative prognosis may present an ethical dilemma for American health professionals, who are used to disclosing a full and truthful diagnosis. However, when treating patients from the Middle East, it is more humane and culturally appropriate to present a poor prognosis gradually and to incorporate it within the context of other information and events. Patients who are told about a fatal illness often give up hope.

Death and Dying

In instances of a grave illness, the family can serve as both a buffer and a clearing-house for information, which it can then "filter" down to the patient in small, digestible bits that may be communicated nonverbally rather than verbally. In general, there is a belief that to speak of death is to bring it about. Therefore, once the caregiver gives a grave diagnosis to family members, it should not be discussed again. It is also inappropriate to suggest a visit from a religious official prior to death because to predict and plan for death prior to the event is believed to take fate out of the hands of Allah. Because hope is kept alive until the last moment, family and friends will not show their grief at the bedside of a dying patient. They will gather around the patient to give him or her hope. Grieving is postponed until after death and may be accompanied by loud wailing. To Muslims, death is preordained and life is considered but a preparation for eternal life. Death is to be accepted as an expression of "the will of Allah."

The length of mourning is specifically stated in the Qur'an. Mourning of family and relatives is limited to three days, while a wife may mourn for her husband for a period of four months and ten days.

ARAB PATIENTS

The majority of Middle Easterners living in the United States are Arab Americans from one of the 22 Arabic-speaking countries that stretch from Morocco to the Persian Gulf. Nearly 82 percent are U.S. citizens whose ancestry can be traced to one of five major groups: Lebanese (47 percent), Syrians (15 percent), Egyptians (9 percent), Palestinians (6 percent), or Iraqis (3 percent). There are Arab Americans living in all 50 states, with 66 percent living in large cities such as Los Angeles, Detroit, and New York. The largest Arab American community is in Dearborn, Michigan, where Arab Americans make up 20 percent of the population. While about 90 percent of all Arabs are Muslims, only 23 percent of Arab Americans are Muslims. According to Zogby International (2001), 90 percent of the first wave (1870–WWII) of Arab immigrants to the United States were Christians who came to flee persecution in the Middle East. However, with recent immigration, Muslim Arabs are the fastest growing subgroup in the Arab American community. At its current rate of growth, the Muslim population in the United States will surpass the Jewish population by the year 2010, making Islam the country's second largest religion.

Educational attainment is highly valued among Arabs—about one-third hold a bachelor's degree and about 15 percent hold a graduate degree. While almost half of the adult population speak a language other than English at home, only 10 percent feel that they do not speak English well.

Keys to Successful Relationships with Arab Patients

1. *Whenever possible, match the patient and caregiver by gender.* Interacting with caregivers of the opposite gender may prove embarrassing and stressful. When having to deal with a medical professional of the opposite sex, the patient may refuse to disclose personal information and may be reluctant to disrobe for a physical examination.

2. *Reveal bad news in stages as part of other information* and ask a family spokesperson (usually the oldest male) to be present.

3. *Do not expect future planning in issues of childbirth and death.* Arab Americans believe that these events are controlled by the will of Allah and that any attempt to plan ahead can be interpreted as an attempt to predict or usurp Allah's will.

4. *Respect a patient's concerns regarding the source of an organ, the ingredients in a medication, or the content of a treatment.* Remember that there may be strong objections to the insertion of a pig's valve or organ into a Muslim patient, the ingestion of a cough medicine or other medication with an alcohol base, or the use of insulin derived from a pig.

5. *Don't try to force the patient to remain autonomous and take responsibility for decision making.* In Arab culture the family's role is to indulge the sick person and take responsibilities off his or her shoulders.

6. *Don't be surprised if the patient or his or her family chooses the most intrusive treatment out of a number of options.* Arabs tend to believe that the more intrusive a medical intervention is, the more effective it is—for example, in cases of cancer, surgical removal is preferred over radiation or chemotherapy.

Major Health Problems and Concerns of Arab Americans

Hypertension, high cholesterol levels, diabetes, and other health conditions associated with diet are common to Arab Americans. As with immigrants from other countries whose traditional diets are nutritionally balanced, with only a minimum of meats and a high level of fruits, vegetables, and unprocessed grains, these conditions tend to worsen with the length of time an Arab immigrant has been in the United States. Another contributing factor is that life in an urban environment tends to be more sedentary than life was in the home country. Because of cultural stigmas attached to admitting to stress or personal problems, psychological help is often rejected. There is also a tendency to ignore or cover up physical health problems for fear that an admission of poor health might hurt their children's chance of marriage.

Traditional Beliefs about the Causes of Illness

Germ theory is usually accepted by most members of Arab cultures. However it exists alongside of a sometimes stronger belief in the evil eye, bad luck, emotional and spiritual distress, winds and drafts, a lack of balance in "hot" and "cold" (see below), inadequate diet, and exposure of one's stomach during sleep as possible causes for physical illness. Mental illness is thought to be caused by sudden fears, the wrath of Allah, or Allah's will. Mental health care is usually only sought after all family and community resources have been exhausted.

"Hot" and "Cold" Theory of Illness (Adapted from the Humoral Theory)

The humoral theory of disease described in ancient Greek texts is the basis of traditional Islamic medicine. Many aspects of life are divided into four: the year is divided into four seasons; matter into fire, air, earth, and water; the body into black bile, blood, phlegm, and yellow bile; and the environment into "hot," "cold," "moist," and "dry." Each illness is treated with the opposite humor—for example, a "hot" disease is treated with a "cold" therapy, a "wet" illness with a "dry" therapy, and so forth. Cupping, cautery, and phlebotomy are also used, although special prayers or foods such as honey, dates, olive oil, and salt are preferred to these approaches.

Arabs attribute illnesses such as headaches, colds, flu, and other bodily aches and pains to extreme shifts from hot to cold and vice versa. For this reason, Arab American parents may overdress their children—even as a preventive against a possible change in the weather. A feverish patient is often covered with many layers of clothing and blankets as a means of maintaining body heat.

Foods are also classified as either "hot" or "cold," and it is believed that the digestive system has to be given the opportunity to adjust to a "hot" or "cold" food before introducing its opposite. Therefore, there is an effort to avoid eating "hot" and "cold" foods during the same meal. "Hot" and "cold" do not necessarily correspond to the temperature of the food. For example, honey and walnuts are considered "hot" foods, while cucumbers and yogurt are considered "cold" foods. An inadequate diet is believed to cause weakness or illness; thus a physically robust person is considered healthier than a thin person.

Supernatural Powers

The evil eye, the powers of jealous people, and supernatural powers such as the devil and *jinn* (evil spirits) are all part of the Muslim religion. The gaze of an envious person gives one the evil eye and is believed to upset the victim's natural balance. Children, especially newborns, are thought to be very susceptible to this, and amulets such as blue beads and figures involving the number 5 are often pinned to the infant's clothing. The devil is thought responsible for unacceptable wishes and acts. In this way, those who experience them can blame them on the devil rather than themselves. It is interesting to note that the Arabic word for insanity, *jenun*, is derived from the word *jinn*.

Causes of Genetic Defects

Arab Americans may attribute the genetic defect of a child to the wrath of Allah, Allah's will, or as Allah's test of endurance for the parents. While religious beliefs require the acceptance and care of these children, the family may try to isolate themselves or hide the defective child. These children are usually cared for at home rather than in an institution. Genetic counseling may also be refused because it is thought to involve tampering with the will of Allah.

Lack of Preventive Care

While it is common for Arab Americans to seek care when symptoms of illness or disease occur, it is less common for them to seek preventive care. This may be because of an Arab reluctance to plan ahead and because of the fear that to "talk about illness is to make it happen." This lack of preventive care is also seen in pediatric clinics that tend to be used by Arab American parents as a place to take children to treat accidents or injuries rather than for child wellness measures. Because male children are preferred, there has been some evidence in poorer families that boys are better nourished than girls.

Attitudes toward Fertility and Birth Control

Due to the popular belief that "Allah decides the size of the family," there are formal Islamic rules regarding the treatment of infertility and birth control. The value placed upon the family and the belief that children are a means of strengthening the family favor high fertility. In fact, among Arab women, infertility can lead to rejection and divorce. Although Islam condones treatment for infertility, the approved methods are limited to artificial insemination of the woman and IVF using the husband's sperm. The use of the sperm of another man is forbidden because it is considered adulterous.

Procreation is considered the purpose of marriage; therefore irreversible forms of birth control such as vasectomy and tubal ligation are forbidden. They are labeled as *haram,* or absolutely unlawful, by Islamic jurists. Abortion is also considered *haram* unless the pregnancy involves the question of legitimacy, presents a threat to the woman's life, or may risk a genetic disorder. Although unwanted pregnancies are sometimes aborted covertly, they are often left to a hope for miscarriage.

Childbearing Taboos and Practices

The cravings of the pregnant woman are satisfied because of a belief that she, or the unborn child, may develop a birthmark in the shape of the unsatisfied craving. While the pregnant woman is indulged by all, the preference for a male child often creates stress for mothers who have no sons. Women who are carrying "high" are believed to be bearing a girl, while women who are carrying "low" are believed to be carrying a boy. Practices that may adversely influence the growth of the fetus may include the habit of giving the "best" food to one's husband or children, the consumption of large quantities of olive oil, and the failure of the woman to stop smoking or limit the intake of caffeine.

Delivery is considered woman's business, and in Arab countries home deliveries with the help of a midwife or neighbors is common. One source reported that Iraqi immigrants living in Detroit tended to follow this same practice. Women openly express pain during labor, but do not ordinarily accept breathing and relaxation techniques. Epidural and spinal anesthesia are often refused because of the fear that it may injure the child.

As in many other cultures, there exists a belief that air may enter a postpartum woman and cause illness if she bathes. There is also a belief that a mother's milk is thinned by washing the breasts. The belief that the postpartum woman must have complete rest in order to recover from the ordeals of labor may delay breast-feeding for two or three days. It is also often believed that nursing at birth causes "colic" pain for the mother and that this condition of the mother can make the baby dumb. Special foods, such as lentil soup, are often given to the mother to increase her milk production, and special teas are drunk to flush and cleanse her body.

It is customary to wrap the baby's stomach at birth to protect the child from cold or wind that may enter the child's body through the stomach. Sometimes the Muslim "call to prayer" is whispered into the baby's ear. Circumcision of the male child is required by Muslim law.

When postpartum depression occurs, female family members assume the woman's responsibilities toward the children and the rest of the family. The mother is simply told that she needs more rest and help.

Response to Pain

Arabs feel that pain is harmful and should be controlled. Confidence in Western medicine leads to the anticipation of immediate relief from pain after surgery. Many Arab patients are often confused and disappointed by the discomfort that often occurs postoperatively. In addition, many Arabs believe that complete bed rest is necessary for a fast and full recovery and may, therefore, be noncompliant with postoperative ambulatory regimes.

Pain is expressed more freely in the presence of the family than in the presence of caregivers. Therefore conflicts often arise when nurses assess that a particular dose of pain medication is adequate, but the patient's family demands the administration of stronger doses of medication.

Somatization of Mental Illness

Because mental illness carries a social stigma, the mentally ill Arab patient is likely to present with abdominal pain, lassitude, anorexia, shortness of breath, and a variety of other vague symptoms. Patients are likely to insist upon tonics, vitamins, or medications for these physical symptoms and refuse medications for psychological problems. Even when a diagnosis of mental illness is accepted, the use of somatic medications rather than psychotherapy is preferred.

Spirituality and Healthcare Practices

In addition to the importance of family, the Muslim's affiliation with his or her particular religious sect forms an important part of his or her personal identity. To Muslims, faith means submission to Allah in preparation for the afterlife by fulfilling the duties of the Qur'an, which are (1) declaration of faith, (2) prayer five times daily, (3) almsgiving, (4) fasting during Ramadan, and (5) the completion in one's lifetime of a pilgrimage to Mecca.

A devout Muslim patient may request that his or her bed or chair be turned toward Mecca and that he or she be provided with a bowl for religious cleansing or ablution before prayer. Prayer is not acceptable unless the Muslim's body, clothing, and place of prayer are clean.

Muslims are required to eat wholesome food and abstain from eating pork, drinking alcohol, or taking illicit drugs. They are expected to be conscious of hygiene, practice moderation in all activities, and remain faithful in adversity by maintaining faith in Allah's mercy and compassion.

Illness is often viewed as a punishment for one's failings, since Allah is considered merciful and compassionate by providing a vehicle for repentance and gratitude. One accepts one's fate as the will of Allah. Euthanasia and suicide are forbidden because they tamper with Allah's will.

Blood Transfusions and Organ Donation

Islamic jurists have established regulations regarding blood transfusions and organ donations. In general, these practices are widely accepted. A dying person and/or his or her family may give permission for the harvesting of organs after death. However, it is not permissible to take an organ from a living person because of the assumption of certain death, the time of which is known only to Allah.

Death and Dying

A dying patient's bed is often turned east to face Mecca. Family and friends may also read to the patient from the Qur'an (Koran). Sections stressing hope and acceptance are particularly favored. After death, the body is washed three times by a Muslim of the same sex and then wrapped in white material and buried as soon as possible. All body orifices are closed and slightly packed with cotton in order to prevent bodily fluids (considered unclean) from escaping. Traditionally, the grave must be made of brick or lined in cement and must face Mecca. Prayers are said at the grave by men, while women who are not close relatives or the deceased's wife gather at the home to recite verses from the Qur'an. These women do not attend the burial. Cremation is not practiced and autopsy is not usually approved out of respect for the dead and a feeling that the body should not be mutilated. Autopsy for forensic reasons or for scientific research and instruction is allowed.

EGYPTIAN PATIENTS

Although Egyptians are Arabs, their language is a distinct dialect and some of their health beliefs and practices differ from those of other Arab groups.

Health Problems and Concerns Common to Members of Egyptian Culture

1. *Parasitic diseases*. Many Egyptians suffer from parasitic diseases. The most common is *schistosoma mansoni* or *schistosoma haematobium*. In human hosts, the female worm expels the eggs, which flow with the blood and become lodged in the liver or urinary tract. The body, which treats the eggs as foreign matter, surrounds the eggs with granular tissue. Some of the results are cirrhosis, liver failure, portal hypertension, esophageal varices, bladder cancer, and renal failure. Another prevalent parasitic disease is filariasis.

2. *Infectious diseases*. Egyptians have one of the highest rates of blindness in the world. Trachoma and other acute eye infections affect 5 percent of the rural population and 2 percent of the urban population. Other infectious diseases include typhoid and paratyphoid fevers, streptococcal disease, rheumatic fever, and tuberculosis. Egyptian American patients who test positive for TB should be questioned regarding a history of BCG injection.

3. *"Modern diseases."* Egyptian immigrants to the United States are likely to become victims of the host of "modern diseases" now affecting Egypt. Some of these are obesity, hypertension, lower back pain, and cardiovascular diseases resulting from stress, obesity, and lack of exercise. Type 2 diabetes, another more recent disease affecting Egyptians, is likely to be exacerbated by obesity.

4. *Thalassemia*. Egyptians are at genetic risk for *b*-thalassemia. This can be detected through carrier screening and prenatal diagnosis.

High-Risk Behaviors of Egyptian Americans

Lack of exercise. Although the importance of regular exercise has recently been publicized in Egypt, exercise is not part of the lifestyle of adult Egyptians or Egyptian Americans. A sedentary lifestyle based upon overindulgence in food has contributed to premature deaths due to massive heart failure.

Diet. Food is an essential part of the Egyptian social system, and Egyptians develop trust through sharing a meal together. Traditional food is rich and high in fat, sodium, and sugar. Because food is associated with health, many Egyptian Americans believe that the more food one eats, the greater one's potential for health. This causes parents and relatives to overfeed their children. Overeating is also encouraged by other beliefs. Food is associated both with the ability of the head of the family to feed his family, and with caring and nurturing. Thus families take pride in the amount of food made available to their family, and mothers and wives display their pride with elaborate cooking of family meals. Food is also considered a demonstration of generosity and giving, and thus the offering and sharing of food demonstrate friendship.

In Egypt, meat dishes were accompaniments to the main vegetable dishes. In the United States, this custom has been reversed. The Egyptian American meal consists of one or more meat dishes with accompanying vegetables and rice. The drinking of tea apart from meals became popular during British rule; however, unlike the English, most Egyptians sweeten their tea with two or three teaspoonsful of sugar.

Some Egyptian Americans avoid drinking water and fluids with meals because they believe that all liquids displace the volume available for solid nutrients or dilute the stomach "juices," making digestion difficult and causing indigestion.

Stomach and intestinal problems such as heartburn, flatulence, constipation, hemorrhoids, and fecal impaction may be caused by limited roughage in the diet, lack of fluids, and rapid consumption of foods. Because Egyptian Americans place great stress on the need for regularity, they tend to push and strain to achieve a bowel movement.

Family Planning, Pregnancy, and Childbearing Practices

Birth control and family planning are never advocated before the birth of the first child, because no Egyptian family is considered complete before a child is born. While the desirable family size in urban Egypt is three or four children, the majority of Egyptian Americans desire a family comprised of two to three children. Families are under stress until their first child is born. Women are threatened with the possibility of divorce if they don't conceive during the first year of marriage—even if the husband is the cause of temporary or permanent infertility. Although in Egypt childbearing is considered woman's business, some acculturated Egyptian American men come in conflict with this cultural principle by participating in the birthing experience. Although Arab culture prohibits bathing or washing one's hair during the 40-day postpartum period, Egyptian American women tend to respond positively to patient education that offers a sound rationale for bathing and information that dispels the fear of infection. During the postpartum period women are expected to refrain from any sexual activity.

The Double Marriage Ceremony

Egyptian American Muslims participate in two marriage ceremonies—one is a religious ceremony performed by the *Imam* and the other is a social ceremony that involves the celebration by family and friends. While both ceremonies may be performed on the same day, the man and woman are not expected to sleep together until after the social ceremony. If the couple separates prior to the social ceremony, it is as if a divorce has taken place. Egyptian American Christians are married by a single religious ceremony.

Shopping for Quality Medical Care

In Egypt, medical care is free or available at a low cost. However, it is believed that good medical care can only be obtained by shopping, bargaining, and negotiation. Egyptian Americans try to join an HMO or purchase health insurance. Some have to postpone the purchase of these services until they achieve financial security. When a health problem develops, family members and friends are usually consulted prior to a health professional. Once they do enter the health system, Egyptian Americans tend to demand immediate, personalized attention. They believe in the value of medical tests and expect to be given medical regimens and prescriptions. They prefer to be given medications and injections but tend to be skeptical of medical advice involving weight reduction, exercise, and diet restrictions. Self-medication is often practiced, and the Egyptian American's medicine cabinet is often filled with antibiotics, tranquilizers, sleeping pills, and pain medications. These are often shared with other family members and friends. Because many of the medications familiar to Egyptian immigrants are unavailable in the United States without prescription, they are often brought from Egypt by family and friends. Intramuscular vitamin injections are preferred over vitamin pills. In Egypt, vitamin B-complex injections and iron supplements are common forms of self-medication.

The American system of meticulous diagnostic approaches may be viewed by some Egyptian immigrant patients as proof of lack of expertise or knowledge. The patient, therefore, may shop around for a physician who lives up to their cultural expectations of a quick, authoritative diagnosis. Others may interpret the need for tests and other resources as an indication of the gravity of their illness.

Gender-Based Preferences

Egyptian Americans who immigrated to the United States before the wave of Islamic fundamentalism may not make gender an important consideration in the choice of a healthcare provider. Later immigrants will prefer providers of the same gender.

IRANIAN PATIENTS

The people. Although Iranians come from the geographic area of the world referred to as the Middle East, they are not Arabs. They are of Indo-European origin and their primary language is Farsi or Persian rather than Arabic. Iran is an extremely heterogeneous country, with nearly half of the country belonging to other ethnic and linguistic groups. Some of the other languages common to Iran are Turkish, Armenian, Baluchi, and Kurdish. French is used as the language of culture and English as the language of business.

Although Iranians came to the United States as students and professionals, with some remaining, as early as the 1950s, and even more in the 1970s, the largest number of Iranian immigrants came after 1979. They came as a result of the Islamic revolution—some for personal and economic reasons, but many as political exiles and forced migrants. Between 1980 and 1990, an estimated 800,000 Iranians of very diverse social, religious, and economic backgrounds immigrated to the United States. Some of these immigrants are either religious or secular Shi'ite Muslims, Sunni Muslims, Jews, Christians (Armenians and Nestorians), Baha'is, and Zoroastrians. Iranian immigrants may be of the university-educated middle class and include physicians, pharmacists, nurses, engineers, professors, and lawyers. Others may be grammar-school-educated merchants and artisans. Some were able to bring their own money and start businesses in the United States; others lost all their resources upon leaving Iran.

Although Iranians share many cultural, health/illness, and illness-prevention practices with Arab peoples, a number of these are unique to those who emigrated from Iran. The most important of these are discussed below.

Health Problems and Concerns Common to Members of Iranian Culture

In Iran, there exist a number of health problems related to underdevelopment, such as protein and vitamin deficiency, hepatitis A and B, and rising rates of TB and syphilis. Other problems caused by intrafamily marriages, such as epilepsy, blindness, anemia, hemophilia, and birth defects, have decreased due to an increased public awareness of these dangers. Thalassemia, once prevalent in northern and eastern provinces, is being addressed through premarital screening. Other common problems are vitamin B_{12} or folic acid deficiencies and Mediterranean glucose-6-phosphate dehydrogenase deficiency.

Traditional Health Beliefs and Practices

Traditional Iranian health beliefs are strongly influenced by the same humoral medical beliefs described in the previous sections. When someone feels ill, he is first asked whether he has eaten something that did not agree with his *mezaj* (personal humoral temperament). If not, other causes are explored.

Iranian Definitions of Health and Illness

Iranians view health as both an absence of disease and the ability to cope successfully with life. This concept involves a dynamic relationship between the individual and the environment. Accordingly, health cannot be achieved through any preplanned schedule of diet, exercise, and therapy, but is, instead, a way of life. Because Iranians accept both biomedical and cultural illness categories, the body is viewed in relation to the total environment, which includes Allah, the supernatural, and society.

Responsibility for Healthcare

Many Iranians use a combination of humoral, Islamic, and modern biomedical approaches to both cure and prevent illness. Often they will seek advice about herbal remedies from elders. Herbal remedies are primarily used to relieve symptoms. When they seek biomedical advice, they tend to expect immediate relief or cures. They may shop around for a physician whom they like or who offers them hope for an immediate or complete cure. Iranians watch their diets to promote health. They are especially careful about ingredients and food preparation. They practice self-medication with prescriptions, over-the-counter medicines, and herbal remedies. They may also adjust the dosage of prescribed medications—especially when finances are a problem. Because of prior overuse of antibiotics, a first generation antibiotic may not be strong enough for an Iranian.

In Iranian culture, the sick person is expected to transfer the responsibility for care into the hands of close family and friends. This may be misinterpreted by American caregivers as a lack of desire for recovery. One approach the health professional can take is to encourage family members to administer appropriate care to the sick person.

Nutrition, Diet, and Health

As for other people from the Middle East, food is a symbol of hospitality. The presentation of Iranian dishes (which usually take hours to prepare) involves a pleasing mixture of colors, textures, and ingredients. The freshness of foods is important, and canned, frozen, and fast foods are avoided because they are believed to have less nutritional value and to contain preservatives that can be harmful to health. Tea is served with every meal, and fresh fruit and leafy green vegetables and fresh herbs are important features of the Iranian diet.

Misuse of Alcohol

Although the Muslim religion prohibits the consumption of alcohol, many Iranians are not religious and drink socially. A low level of acculturation in the United

States and a sense of helplessness experienced by some Iranian immigrants, especially men, sometimes lead to misuse of alcohol in an attempt to demonstrate an ability to "hold their liquor" as a means of showing their masculinity.

Fertility, Pregnancy, and Childbearing Practices

According to Iranian tradition, the man contributes his seed and the woman provides the vessel in which the seed grows.

Menstrual blood is considered ritually unclean and physically polluting, and menstruating women are forbidden to touch holy objects or to have intercourse. Women are not supposed to exercise or shower excessively during menstruation because they are thought to be fragile and susceptible to hemorrhage. At the end of menses, and prior to participating in any religious rituals, women are expected to wash and purify themselves. Pregnancy soon after marriage is considered desirable, not only to make the family complete, but also because women believe that pregnancy makes them healthier. This notion is tied to the belief that excess menstrual blood "clogs the body" prior to pregnancy. This excess is reduced during the nine months that menses does not occur and the remainder is discharged during the birth of their first child.

Birth Control

Because Iranians believe it is necessary for the woman to discharge blood monthly, Iranians discourage the use of any form of birth control that decreases the menstrual blood flow. Some women have also complained that these methods give them such symptoms as heart palpitation.

Prior to the revolution in 1979, birth control was rarely used in rural areas because children ensured the financial success of the family. After 1979, contraception was discouraged because of the Islamic belief that children are Allah's blessing. One traditional method of birth control was prolonged breast-feeding. In instances of infertility, the woman was always blamed. It was thought that fertility depended upon the health of the uterus, and home remedies focused upon ways of improving the health of the uterus. The desired number of children for an urban educated Iranian family is three to four children in Iran, but only two to three children for Iranians living in the United States.

Childbirth

The cravings of a pregnant woman are thought to represent the need of the fetus for those foods. Failure to satisfy these needs is believed to cause the child to be born with a birthmark in the shape of the food that was craved.

Sexual intercourse is allowed until the last month of pregnancy. Because heavy work is believed to cause miscarriage, the pregnant woman receives a great deal of help and support from female relatives—including relief from household chores from the sixth month of pregnancy through after the birth. During pregnancy the woman avoids fried foods and those that are believed to cause gas. Fruits and vegetables are recommended.

Commonly present during the birthing process is the woman's mother, sister, or aunt. Walking prior to delivery is recommended and Iranian women in the United States are generally agreeable to Lamaze classes. Although in traditional Iranian families the husband is not involved, in the United States Iranian families follow the diverse practices of the dominant culture. Some women involve their husbands fully in the birthing process, with some expressing a preference for natural childbirth and others for medication.

Breast-feeding is usually preferred over bottle-feeding and is mixed with solid food at about 4 to 6 months of age. Breast-feeding may last as long as one year and is not usually mixed with bottle-feeding unless the mother is working outside the home.

Depression

Narahati is the Iranian word for feeling depressed, ill at ease, nervous, inconvenienced, or anxious. Iranians sometimes express the cultural and social losses due to the war and immigration through somatization. Others may manifest it psychologically through either withdrawal or expressions of anger.

Sensitivity is a highly valued trait in Iranian culture. However, the sensitive person can be both socially vulnerable and potentially powerless. *Narahati* is an Iranian word that is used to express undifferentiated and unpleasant emotional and physical feelings. These feelings are expressed verbally or nonverbally in a number of ways. The word is seldom used, though when *narahati* is expressed verbally, the person speaks publicly about his or her troubles and what caused them. More often than not, however, *narahati* is expressed nonverbally through one of the following three ways: (1) silence, quietness, and sulkiness; (2) avoidance of food as a means of withdrawing from social interaction; or (3) crying (more prevalent among women than among men).

Often *narahati* is camouflaged because of a feeling of personal powerlessness, a belief that it connotes fate and, therefore, one can do nothing about it, or a fear that an expression of one's own *narahati* will make someone else *narahati*.

Feelings of anger and sadness are not usually camouflaged. The adjective for angry in Farsi, *asabani,* is derived from the Arabic word *asab*, which means "nerve," rather than "nervous." In other words, it signifies that the nerves are not functioning properly because to be angry is to be out of control. Being out of control could cause personal or familial embarrassment or shame. Anger, in Iranian society, is a somatopsychic phenomenon. It has social causes and very definite social repercussions. However, where anger is considered unacceptable because it disrupts social life, sadness is accepted as a profound condition. *Ghamgini* is the Iranian word for sorrow or sadness. It cannot be camouflaged because it is visibly displayed on the person's face. This sense of sadness is considered an almost poetic condition in Iranian culture and is thus accepted. It indicates a loss. This can be the loss of a person, one's livelihood, or one's country. It is a private emotion that is publicly expressed.

Narahati and anger are somatized when they cannot be expressed (verbally or nonverbally) in socially appropriate ways. In these cases, the body becomes a metaphor for personal distress. In this way the person can distance himself or herself from personal problems and can be absolved of responsibility for them. Common physical complaints such as chest pains, stomachaches or other digestive problems, and pains in the limbs are acceptably expressed, whereas it is not acceptable to express personal *narahati*.

A description of a disease known in Iranian culture as *kam khun* and its treatment illustrates the way in which Iranian culture views the working of the body somatopsychically rather than psychosomatically. *Kam khun*, or blood deficiency, is the term used by Iranians to describe an ailment that is believed to develop from excessive bleeding from menstruation, an accident, an operation, improper diet, and so forth. Its main symptom is physical weakness. However, because there is not enough blood to nourish the nerves, *asabani* (anger) can result. In Iranian folk medicine, this condition is treated with tonics, infusions, and foods (especially foods high in iron such as liver, lentils, and spinach). In other words, *kam khun* describes an entire range of physical ailments involving weakness, thinness, headaches, and other disorders. It is considered a physical ailment and has physical manifestations.

Suggested Approach to Somatization

Iranian refugees suffer from a variety of physical and somatized ailments such as *kam khun*. These may be expressed in a number of culturally distinctive ways. The Iranian patient may present with complaints of pains in a high-pitched voice, speaking softly and bowing his or her head to show respect for the physician as an educated authority figure. A caregiver who acknowledges the patient's personal and social situation will be better able to establish a trusting relationship with the patient. Although the patient may see no connection between his or her personal problems and the physical pain, it may be helpful to ask the patient about his or her difficulties in adjusting to life in the States. It is also helpful to ask about any herbal remedies that the patient may be taking. Patients should be encouraged to follow the "hot"/"cold" dietary regimen and to continue taking any herbal remedies that will not harm them.

Death and Dying

Iranian patients, regardless of their religious affiliation, tend to oppose the cessation of life support due to the cultural belief that life and death are controlled by Allah. The right to die is not recognized because only Allah can decide when a person will die. However, it is advised that the caregiver make an individual assessment of the family. If death is imminent, the caregiver may try to initiate a discussion with the family spokesperson, suggesting that using mechanical means of life support may itself be usurping Allah's will.

DEVELOPING CULTURAL PERSPECTIVE

1. Why is it taboo among Muslims to speak about death?

2. If you hear a Muslim patient repeating a statement loudly several times, what non-verbal message is that patient communicating? How should you respond?

3. Given a choice between an invasive treatment and a non-invasive treatment, which would an Arab patient be more likely to choose?

4. How does the Middle Eastern concept of "personal space" differ from your concept? How might that make you uncomfortable?

5. How does the Iranian concept of menstruation affect their belief about birth control?

BLENDING PERSPECTIVES

1. How do you communicate the importance of a verbal message? Through tone? Volume? Facial expression? Body language? Choice of words? Do you use the same cues to discern the importance of an incoming verbal message? Are there any modifications you can make to your style to accommodate other cultures?

2. What are the implications of the concept of "fate" or the "will of Allah" upon personal responsibility and decision-making? How might they affect healthcare choices?

Chapter 7

Providing Culture-Sensitive Healthcare to Emigrés from the Former Soviet Bloc Countries of Russia, Bosnia, and Poland

Keys to a Good Professional Relationship

1. *Introduce yourself using your title and family name.* Address all adult patients by their title (Mr., Mrs., Dr., Professor, etc.) and family name. Although many Russian, Polish, and Bosnian family names are difficult to pronounce, an effort to try to pronounce them and a genuine request to be corrected and helped will be greatly appreciated.

2. *Keep in mind that these patients may have been used to a healthcare system that was authoritarian and paternalistic.* Often patients were not told what ailments they had or given an explanation of exactly what treatment they would receive. Cancer, especially, was never mentioned to the patient.

3. *Inform the patient that the nurse is following the physician's orders when performing even a routine procedure such as taking a patient's temperature or blood pressure.* This is because patients and their families may distrust any care or advice given by a nurse and may demand to see the doctor. This distrust stems from the fact that nurses in their countries have no autonomy and are not responsible for any treatment. One way around this is to explain that "Dr. X instructed me to do this and tell you that …"

4. *Young physicians and nurses should not take offense if the patient appears not to trust them or demands to see a specialist.* In their countries youth is suspect, yet it is considered a breach of confidence or trust to ask for a second opinion. Care given by young resident physicians may be considered inadequate, and specialists equated with senior physicians who are referred to as "professor" in their countries. Older physicians hold higher status in the medical community because age is often equated (especially by older patients) with wisdom, knowledge, and experience. A request for a referral to a specialist is one strategy the patient may use to develop confidence in an unfamiliar medical system.

5. *Explain that in the American healthcare system hospital stays are avoided unless absolutely necessary.* In the former Soviet bloc countries, hospital stays are generally more frequent and last longer than in the United States. Patients may therefore be disturbed by the many treatments that in the United States are routinely offered as outpatient services as well as by the short hospital stays required for surgery or childbirth. Many of the treatments provided by the medical systems in these countries were holistic in nature. In the Soviet system, for example, patients were often sent to a sanatorium or spa for extended stays of up to a month where the treatment consisted of massage, herbal baths, light exercise, and homeopathic and herbal cures. These remedies are used to "remove" the illness.

6. *The purpose and value of a diagnostic test should always be explained carefully.* However, it is not advisable to go into detail about the procedure. Diagnostic tests are used much less frequently in the former Soviet bloc countries than in the United States because they are often scarce and very costly. Physicians in these countries are trained to rely on their examination or diagnostic skills, except in cases where a very serious illness is suspected. Therefore, a patient may either associate a diagnostic test with being seriously ill or discount its value and reliability because it is so readily available. Elderly Russian Jewish patients may even fear that they are being used as guinea pigs for medical experimentation.

7. *When a gift other than money is offered, it is best to accept it graciously after explaining that gifts are not necessary or expected.* This is because salaries for physicians and other healthcare workers are often so low in these countries that some sort of tip or auxiliary payment is expected for attentive care. While ethical standards in the United States require that a monetary gift be politely refused, caregivers should not take offense if one is offered.

8. *Be prepared to accept or prescribe herbal treatments in conjunction with pharmaceutical treatments.* New immigrants may have more confidence in herbal combinations than patent drugs for chronic illnesses because it is believed that too much of any medicine can be poisonous. Physicians in Poland, Russia, and Bosnia often prescribe herbal drugs and treatments prepared by pharmacists who follow the physician's notations on a prescription form. Mt. Zion Hospital, a hospital in San Francisco that served a large Soviet Jewish emigré population in the 1980s, began to use tincture of valerian (8–10 drops taken in a glass of water) to treat this population for symptoms of insomnia or anxiety. While it was never proven scientifically whether results were medicinal or placebo, its long-term effects on patients' complaints were excellent.

9. *Specifically ask patients to bring in any and all of the medications (herbal or other) they are taking when they come into your office or clinic.* Many of the medications given in the United States are unfamiliar, expensive, and/or suspect. Sometimes, medications that are not known or used in the United States are mailed or brought into this country by visitors from the patient's home country. While most of this medication is not intrinsically harmful, it could double the dose of American prescriptions or have negative interactions with them. On the other hand, American "brand-name" over-the-counter drugs such as Bayer Aspirin are extremely popular in the former Soviet bloc countries. These may be requested by brand by relatives at home. Patients may even ask their United States physician for prescriptions for these relatives. This is because they do not understand our stringent regulations about prescribing only to one's own patients.

10. *In cases of obesity, diabetes, heart disease, or high cholesterol, it is important to question patients carefully about their diet.* The cold climates that these patients come from, the poorer quality of meats available and, in most cases,

distances from the sea tended to encourage the consumption of root vegetables (boiled until there are few nutrients left) in stews and soups high in fat content. The traditional diet in countries of the former Soviet bloc consists of a breakfast of bread, tomatoes (when available), and ham and sausage (the sausage category includes salami, jellied tongue, liver sausage, etc.). A large hot meal with potatoes is eaten at midday and cold cuts (again sausage) at night. Although the sequence of meals immigrants eat tends to be shifted to coincide with United States working hours, the diet of newer immigrants often favors these ingredients. It is important to talk to the person responsible for shopping and meals about healthier choices if any member of the family suffers from any of the above problems.

Health Problems and Concerns

1. *Obesity, gallbladder disease, diabetes, elevated cholesterol levels, cardiovascular disease.* Food plays a major part in the rules of hospitality and in many of the religious and cultural traditions in each of the groups from the former Soviet bloc nations. All have a tradition of eating foods that are high in saturated fat content. The cold, hard winters that all regions share have produced similarities in the traditional diets of the Russian, Ukrainian, Bosnian, and Polish immigrants to the United States. Despite the fact that Russian Jews and Muslim Bosnians are forbidden to eat pork—a common meat in the Polish diet—the need to preserve food without refrigeration has made dried sausage and the pickling (high salt content) of meats, fish, and vegetables popular. Russian Jews substitute chicken fat for the cooking lard used in Polish cooking as well as for the butter used on the large quantities of bread that are consumed by each group. Long, cold winters make root vegetables more available than leafy green vegetables, and their use in stews and heavy soups means that most of the nutrients are cooked out. While it is customary for Russian Jews to eat chicken (which is often boiled with the skin on) and Poles to eat carp (often boiled or fried in lard) on Friday nights, the fat content and the overcooking of vegetables is probably similar in both cultures. This high-fat diet, combined with the fact that regular exercise is not a cultural norm, especially for older members, contributes to the propensity for obesity, diabetes, and heart disease.

2. *Lung disease and cancer as a result of smoking and pollution.* Many older Russian Jews, Ukrainians, and Poles are heavy smokers. Those who come from large urban areas often display many of the respiratory problems caused by air pollution produced by large factories. The immigrants from Poland and the Russian areas around Chernobyl also need to be checked regularly for the many cancer-producing aftereffects of nuclear fallout.

3. *Alcoholism.* Although alcoholism is not a frequent problem with Russian Jews or Pentecostal Christians (who are forbidden to use alcohol or tobacco), it is a long-standing problem of Ukrainian and Polish Americans. Although most Muslims are forbidden to drink, most Bosnian Muslims consider themselves Europeans first and Muslims second and may drink alcohol. While alcoholism has been mentioned as a frequent problem in the former Yugoslavia and drinking alcohol is permitted by the Bosnian Muslim church, there is nothing in the literature to indicate that alcoholism is a major health problem with any of the three major religious groups in Bosnia.

4. *Somatization of mental illness.* Because mental illness is considered a stigma in most countries of the former Soviet bloc, the depression and stress that are often caused by the inherent problems of immigration, such as having to deal with a strange culture, physical environment, and language, are often channeled into physical complaints.

RUSSIAN PATIENTS

Healthcare in Russia under the Former Soviet Union

In spite of an initial idealism of equality, the communists inherited the Russian feudal expectancy of being cared for by "our father the Czar." Although there was little real confidence in the State as an institution, there was always an underlying expectation that the "father" or authoritarian state system was supposed to care for one. The health system in Soviet Russia was organized around regional clinics. When one became sick one would stay in bed and wait for a medical aid, called a *feldsher*, to provide care. (This type of medical aid also exists in Poland. In Polish the name for the aid is the same but takes on the Polish spelling, *felczer*.) Clinics were open a set number of hours and physicians worked a fixed shift. If the physician didn't have time to see all the patients by the end of the shift, he or she simply left and the patients had to come back the next day. Appointments weren't maintained so patients tended to arrive early (or very late with an "emergency"), complain loudly, and repeatedly remind the nurses that they were present.

Many Russian immigrant patients are frequently viewed as loud and complaining by caregivers in the United States, who soon come to suspect that they are exaggerating their pain or symptoms. Tolerance of these unpleasant traits may be improved by an understanding that the patients come from a system in which it was definitely a case of "the person who makes the loudest noise" getting the best (or often the only) treatment. A complaint of severe chest pain was often the only way to get seen, and this complaint was often used as a means of beating an otherwise uncaring, unresponsive system.

In general, healthcare resources were very scarce and healthcare was provided under poor conditions. Drug and equipment supplies were erratic. By 1990, even aspirin and penicillin were difficult to obtain and infant mortality was extremely high. With the collapse of the Soviet Union and the attempt to switch to a market economy, many more Western prescription drugs became available over the counter at pharmacies and even sidewalk markets.

In spite of the lack of finances and facilities in the former Soviet Union, the concept in the United States of short hospital stays is very different from the practices of most former Soviet bloc nations. One report published by the *Western Journal of Medicine* in 1982 stated that one in every four Russians was admitted for a hospital stay every year, and the average length of each hospital stay was 15 days. In the former Soviet Union, a hospital was commonly viewed as a place to queue up for tests and treatments. According to Grabbe (see Appendix C), the Soviet Union had triple the number of hospital beds and double the number of doctors per capita as in the United States. Caregivers' pay was so poor that extra pay was expected—and given—for even routine nursing care such as bathing patients or administering pain medication in a timely fashion. Physicians regularly received hard-to-get goods and extra monetary "gifts" from the patient and the patients' families.

Forms of Treatment

Folk medicine was not only tolerated but often prescribed by Soviet bloc physicians. Treatment often, therefore, consisted of a blend of Western medicine, folk medicine, and the use of natural resources such as water, fresh air, minerals, and sun. Baby urine and animal bile (sold in pharmacies) placed on a cloth and wrapped around an "offending" limb was commonly used to treat arthritic joints. Use of home remedies was prevalent. In Kazakhstan, for example, horse fat was used for bursitis and skin wounds, and wrapping one's back in dog hide was a treatment for back pain.

While birth control pills are now more readily available, during the Soviet period, the principal form of contraception was abortion or folk cures such as drinking vodka and then taking a sauna.

Immigration from the Soviet Union to the United States

The majority of immigrants to the United States from the former Soviet Union during the twentieth century have been Jews. The first major wave of immigrants from Russia came between 1881 and 1914. About half of them were Jews. The next major wave came between 1920 and 1922 to escape the communist rule. The third occurred just after World War II. The most recent immigration occurred in the 1970s when the Soviet government permitted Jews to move to Israel, and many used their move there as a stepping stone to joining relatives in the United States. Between 1971 and 1991, about 181,000 Russian Jews came to the United States. Statistics show that fully two-thirds of those who emigrated from Russia in the year 1991 were Jews. The majority of the Soviet emigrés who were not Jews belonged to the Pentecostal Church. It is estimated that 2,000 Pentecostal Christians emigrated to the United States from the Soviet Union between 1971 and 1991.

According to the 2000 U.S. Census, there were 624,000 people from the former Soviet Union living in the United States. In 2003, Russia ranked tenth among the top twenty countries of origin for immigrants to the United States.

While many of the Russian Jews who immigrated to the United States after World War I were "Jewish" by culture, many were not Jewish by religion. After the Bolshevik Revolution of 1917, Jews and other religious groups were "discouraged" from following their religious practices. Thus, many of these immigrants neither go to synagogue nor know any Yiddish or Hebrew.

The elderly. Immigration from Russia was by entire families, rather than by individuals. During the Soviet period, elderly, "unproductive" citizens were not permitted to remain in Russia if no young, working adults were willing to stay to care for them. Thus, many of the immigrants coming to the United States came for the "good of the children" or because they were forced to come. Of the Russian Jews who came to the United States in 1991, 20 percent were over the age of 65. Not only did these immigrants suffer many of the illnesses commonly associated with old age, but these illnesses were more pronounced than those of most elderly citizens in the United States due to the many years when all Russians suffered from lack of food (especially fruits and vegetables) and adequate medical care.

An Urban, Highly Educated Group of "Survivors"

The Russian Jews tend to come from very large urban areas. Although many are highly educated (there is a 100 percent literacy rate), age, differences in professional accreditation standards, and lack of language proficiency have kept them from finding jobs or job satisfaction in the United States.

Because there has traditionally been much prejudice against Jews in Russia, those who have survived revolution and two world wars prior to having emigrated to the United States have had to develop great strength and fortitude. They are primarily people who learned early in life to demand loudly and continuously as a means of coping successfully with the Soviet system. These traits have been carried to the United States with them and have earned them a less-than-popular reputation as patients in the U.S. healthcare system. Caregivers have often described Russian patients' behavior as being manipulative and abrasive. They are often suspected of exaggerating symptoms that impair normal functioning or somatizing minor complaints in order to obtain more immediate attention.

Health Problems and Concerns Common to Members of Russian Culture

1. *Lifestyle and longevity.* The lifestyle many Russian emigrés have brought with them is not conducive to health maintenance. The majority of people in the former Soviet Union tend to follow a diet high in fat and low in green vegetables and to have no tradition of regular exercise.

   Although in the Soviet Union liquor has contributed to a high level of liver disease, malnutrition, and cardiovascular disease, as well as mortality from accidents, poisons, and injuries, the majority of emigrés from the former Soviet Union have been Jews and Pentecostal Christians. Pentecostal Christians are forbidden to use alcohol or tobacco, and Jewish culture has always frowned upon the use of alcohol not related to religious rituals. Although few Jews who grew up during the Soviet period are religious because religious training was forbidden and atheism was encouraged, many dietary habits and restrictions are followed for cultural if not religious reasons. Pork is forbidden and the kosher home, which also forbids the use of butter (a dairy product) with meats, has traditionally used chicken fat both as a substitute for cooking and to spread on bread. Most families in the Soviet Union were three-generation families. The elderly served the important functions of scavenging for scarce food staples, standing on lines to purchase goods, cooking, and caring for children so both parents could work. Traditional eating habits have been passed on by this older generation.

   Longevity is also affected by the frequency of abortion in women of childbearing age. This is due to the fact that, in the Soviet Union, it was very difficult to obtain effective contraceptive devices. Women have therefore had to rely heavily on abortion—often performed as late as the twelfth week of pregnancy.

2. *Life expectancy.* Since a substantial number of emigrés arrived in the United States when they were already over 65 and others will now be over 65, it is important to note that according to 1990 figures, the life expectancy for men in the Soviet Union ranged from 68.0 years for men in Georgia to 60.7 years for men in Turkmenistan, compared to 71.8 years for men in the United States according to the 1994 Census. For women, life expectancy ranged from 75.7 years in Georgia to only 68.8 years in Turkmenistan, as opposed to 78.8 years for women born in the United States. These shorter life-expectancy figures can probably be attributed to a combination of factors that includes inadequate healthcare, poor nutrition, and a fairly unhealthy lifestyle. These factors cannot be undone easily through immigration to the United States fairly late in life. Exacerbating these factors is the fact that many older emigrés did not come to the United States out of choice but came "for the good of the children" or because the Soviet Union would not allow them to stay unless younger family members remained in Russia to take care of them.

3. *Women's health.* A study conducted in Israel in the late 1990s (see Remennick, Appendix C) indicated that women from the former Soviet Union rated their health as poorer than that of other immigrants and had a higher prevalence of chronic disease and depression. Nevertheless, they had a lower incidence of visits to specialists. These immigrant women had a strong tendency to neglect most preventive measures and older women (60-plus) had a low level of awareness and preventive practices with regard to breast cancer screening. Soviet data indicate that breast cancer is the most prevalent form of cancer in

Soviet women, followed by cervical cancer. Jewish women, regardless of education and economic status, have a cancer rate higher than the national average. Other risk factors include low fertility and postmenopausal obesity.

BOSNIAN PATIENTS

The people. Bosnia is the only part of the former Yugoslavia that was organized along geographical and historical rather than ethnic lines. Before the Bosnian War (1992–95), the population of Bosnia was diverse. Approximately 44 percent were Muslims, 31 percent Serbs, and 17 percent Croats. There were also small numbers of Gypsies, Albanians, Ukrainians, Poles, and Italians living in Bosnia.

Muslims. The Muslim population tends to be more urban than that of those belonging to Serbian or Croatian groups. This is possibly due to the privileges that Muslims enjoyed during the long Ottoman occupation from the fifteenth to the nineteenth century. Muslim Bosnians are not, as might be expected, descendants of Turks who were left behind when the Ottomans withdrew from the territory. They are actually descendants of Serbian and Croatian Slavs who converted to Islam after the Ottoman conquest of Bosnia in the fifteenth century. Most converts were attracted by the willingness of the Ottomans to recognize them as nobility and/or as a means of avoiding the high taxes and restrictions levied against Christians.

Before the 1878 occupation of Bosnia by Austria, those who lived in Bosnia were classified as being either "Yugoslav," a name that can be translated as "southern Slav," or "Other." The Austrians identified the group geographically as Bosniaks rather than Muslims, Serbs, or Croats in order to avoid any possible territorial claims from either Serbia or Croatia. After World War II, Bosnia became one of the republics of Yugoslavia under the rule of President Tito. It wasn't until the census of 1971 that Muslims gained recognition as a separate ethnic category.

As with the majority of the Bosnian population, most urban Muslims considered themselves Europeans and Bosnians first, and Muslims second. The war has tended to change that by awakening a much greater sense of identification with Muslim culture.

Language. The primary language of Bosnia is Serbo-Croatian. Most of those who speak it as a first language will refer to it as Bosnian. There is also a distinctly local (Bosnian) tongue that is written in the Latin alphabet, rather than the Cyrillic alphabet of Serbo-Croatian. Some population groups speak a Gypsy (Romany) dialect, Albanian, or Ukrainian. Most Bosnians have had some exposure to English or German in school.

Education. A 1996 survey of almost 200 Bosnian refugees to the United States indicated a fairly high degree of education, with 42 percent of this group having completed secondary school in Bosnia and 35 percent having completed university. Among this group, some had been professionals such as physicians, architects, teachers, or social workers, while others had been skilled or unskilled workers. Over 75 percent were employed in unskilled or entry-level positions in the United States.

Geography/climate. Northern Bosnia contains over 70 percent of the cultivated land that existed in the former Yugoslavia. The land becomes more mountainous as one moves south. Western Bosnia is not very fertile.

The capital of Bosnia, Sarajevo, is in the central region of the country. The greatest population density is urban rather than rural. The climate in Bosnia, like much of the surrounding region, is hot and humid in summer while harsh and cold in winter.

Availability and Quality of Healthcare

As in most former Soviet bloc countries, healthcare was free of charge throughout the countries that had been part of Yugoslavia. The quality and standard of care was also considered comparable with that provided in Western Europe. The presence of several international pharmaceutical companies made it fairly easy to obtain medications. In spite of the above, physicians were poorly paid and it was expected that patients and their families offer monetary and material compensation to caregivers as a means of ensuring quality care or to obtain longer periods of "work leave authorization" from district physicians.

Training for nurses in Bosnia was at a trade school rather than a university level, so Bosnian patients may not be familiar with the level of training that nurses receive in the United States. They may not understand why U.S. nurses commonly take a patient's pulse or blood pressure or even give routine medical advice.

Healthcare in prewar Bosnia was divided into three sectors. *Ambulantas,* small community-based clinics, provided both primary care and emergency services. Most patients were sent from there to centralized multidisciplinary clinics or health centers largely staffed by specialists. These sites provided most diagnostic and treatment procedures. The tertiary level of care was provided by teaching hospitals and university medical schools. Thus, most healthcare in prewar Bosnia was provided by specialists, while the primary care physicians played a far less visible or influential role. Even routine women's health procedures such as PAP smears were performed by gynecologists rather than primary care physicians. In general, healthcare was universal and of good quality, although not as technologically advanced as in the United States. The system was easy for patients to maneuver, there was reportedly little or no wait to see a physician, and it was possible to see as many as four physicians in a single day.

Although the Searight study (see Appendix C) only interviewed twelve refugees, all compared the healthcare system in the United States unfavorably with the prewar Bosnian system and complained of confusion and anxiety. Although they recognized the superior technology of the American system, they felt that the hospital stays were too short to provide adequate quality care and that care was less sensitive, impersonal, and overly concerned with efficiency. They expressed the opinion that American caregivers are so engrossed in paperwork and bureaucracy that healthcare in the United States is a business rather than a system to provide care for those in need of it.

Bosnians in the United States

Over 300,000 Bosnian refugees came to the United States during the 1990s as a result of the Balkan wars. As there were already about 80,000 Bosnians (including 2,500 Muslims) living in the Chicago area prior to the war, when Bosnian war refugees started coming to the United States in 1994, the majority came to the Chicago area because of family ties. Now, however, Bosnians have settled throughout the country—many of them in states that previously had very few foreigners. Most of these refugees are older, have experienced significant war-related trauma, and are used to universal healthcare of a fairly high quality.

Social Structure and Family Values

All Bosnians, regardless of religion or ethnic group, place a very high value upon family, strong friendship networks, land, and hospitality. In the family, the husband/father is considered the head of the family, although urbanization and the ability (and need) for the woman to work outside of the home has led to greater shared responsibility in family decision-making. In rural areas, it was common for three generations to live in one household, with the grandparents playing a very active role to free both parents to be able to work in the fields or outside the home. In urban areas, however, the nuclear family system was more common because of the lack of space in urban apartments.

Dating and Marriage

Customs for dating and marriage are much the same for Bosnians as they are for Europeans or Americans, with one exception. Traditionally, Bosnian Muslim newlyweds moved in with the husband's family so that the mother of the groom could "train" the bride to care for her family. For the past 15 years, there has been a high degree of mixed marriages because of the lack of interest given to whether one was a Muslim, Serb, or Croat. One source states that the Bosnians in Minnesota, the majority of whom are Muslim, seem to be marrying at a younger age than they did in Bosnia.

Maternity Care

Children are highly valued and welcomed in most Bosnian families. Birth control devices were severely limited in spite of the fact that there were a number of pharmaceutical companies in the former Yugoslavia. The two most widely used methods of birth control were oral contraceptives and abortion, both to limit the number of children born and to control the length of time between births. It is not unusual for Bosnian refugees in the United States to request assisted abortion as a means of ending unwanted pregnancies. Caregivers are advised to discuss with all women of childbearing age the many options open to women in the United States as a means of controlling and spacing pregnancies.

Bosnian refugees may be surprised and dissatisfied with the attitudes of caregivers toward childbirth. This is because under Bosnian law pregnant working women are given a month of paid leave prior to childbirth and from four months to a year after childbirth. Prior to the war in Bosnia, women remained in the hospital for about 10 days for natural childbirth and up to 14 days for a cesarean birth.

Disclosure of Life-Threatening or Terminal Illness

Caregivers should use extreme caution when discussing a serious illness directly with a patient. As in many places throughout the world, in Bosnia a patient would never be told that he or she had a life-threatening or terminal illness. This would be considered a death sentence—especially if that disease were cancer. The family may be informed but should be consulted regarding just how much information should be revealed to the patient, and in what manner. While caregivers in the United States might consider this a breach of patient/physician confidentiality or a procedure that robs the patient of his or her autonomy, it must be remembered that autonomy and sharing in medical decision-making are fairly unique to the healthcare system in the United States. The Bosnian patient may neither wish to be informed nor be ready to accept information regarding the seriousness of the illness.

Family members will generally want to be present during the final moments of a patient's life.

Traditional Health Beliefs and Practices

The common practice of attempting to cure minor health problems and illnesses with herbs and special foods prior to seeking care at a health facility has been carried to the United States by many Bosnian refugees. The home garden in which herbs are grown is extremely important. This author has been told by a former nurse from Bosnia, who went on to become a teacher of high school biology, that one reason most of the local refugee population strive so hard to own their own piece of land is because of the importance given to the herbs and vegetables grown there. Common remedies include a cabbage leaf pressed to the wound to reduce swelling, a slice of potato or the oil of a plant pressed to the forehead to cure a headache, or a drink made out of boiled parsley for stomachache. These remedies may or may not be discontinued when care by a biomedical physician is sought.

Health Problems and Concerns Common to Members of Bosnian Culture

1. *Emphysema, lung cancer, and cardiovascular disease as a result of smoking.* Many Bosnians, especially men, are heavy smokers and suffer the types of lung and throat problems caused or irritated by cigarette smoke. Now that we know the harm done by secondhand smoke, it is also suggested that caregivers carefully consider not only the harm done to the smoker but also to other members of the family.

2. *Diabetes, high blood pressure, heart disease, and obesity are also health problems.* Food is a major element of family and social gatherings and anyone visiting a Bosnian household will be expected to eat a meal, or at least have a coffee and pastry or a drink with some snacks. A type of coffee known as "Turkish coffee" is also drunk in great quantities (again, primarily by men). This coffee is ground very finely, mixed with one or two teaspoonsful of sugar per small demitasse cup, and boiled. Although one leaves the grounds, some of the grounds are consumed with each cup. Turkish coffee is not only very sweet but is often accompanied by very sweet desserts, contributing to a high sugar intake. Although Bosnians do consume a fairly good quantity of vegetables, they also eat a lot of fatty foods. Their diet, coupled with a lack of a tradition of regular exercise, can be a contributing factor to illness. Other factors have to do with a lack of understanding regarding the need to complete a full cycle of antibiotics. The medication is often discontinued as soon as it brings some relief or because the patient has been told that he cannot drink while on a course of antibiotics.

3. *War trauma and mental health.* There is a strong stigma against mental health problems of any kind in Bosnian culture. This stigma may prevent refugees who have a past history of mental illness from providing this information during a patient history. Mental illness was not discussed outside the family, and the family and/or patient may try to conceal any past or present mental problem from caregivers or refugee organizations because they fear that it will negatively impact their status as refugees.

   When there is a suspicion that a patient may be suffering from posttraumatic stress disorder (PTSD) or depression caused by war-related trauma, the patient and the patient's family should be helped to understand that the healthcare system in the United States is accepting of mental problems and the need for mental health treatment. It is important that a culturally appropriate approach be used when referring a Bosnian patient to the Center for Victims of Torture or to a mental health provider who has special knowledge and experience in the identification and treatment of war-related trauma.

Suggestions for Caregivers of Bosnian Refugees

1. *Try to learn when and under what circumstances the patient came to the United States.* This information is especially important in treating refugees from war-torn areas to help identify or rule out illnesses/diseases that may have their origins in deprivations suffered during the war or that may be caused by post-traumatic stress or depression.

2. *Talk with the patient and/or the patient's family about their most common health practices.* What do they usually do/take if they have a fever, stomachache, or other ailment? Whom do they consult prior to going to a physician? What home remedies do they give or take?

3. *Ask the patient to bring in any and all medications.* These medications should include those that are natural remedies and any brought/sent from Bosnia so the caregiver can determine whether they might interact with medications he or she wishes to prescribe.

4. *Offer patient education about the United States healthcare system (in print and verbally) in Bosnian.* Take special care to inform the patient and his or her family about both the accepting attitude toward mental illness and the forms of treatment available.

POLISH PATIENTS

The people. Poles have a long history of immigration to the United States. Polish immigration can be divided into three major waves—each for a different reason and each involving different segments of the population in Poland. These differences influenced Polish assimilation into American culture and their health beliefs and practices, as well as their needs and expectations of the U.S. healthcare system.

The first wave of Polish immigrants arrived in the United States between 1820 and 1940, comprising a group of approximately 400,000. Those who arrived between the late 1800s and 1914 are considered *chlebam* or "bread" immigrants because they emigrated for economic reasons. Most were illiterate, unskilled laborers who gathered in urban areas and worked in low-paying jobs.

The second major wave of immigrants arrived after World War II. They were primarily political activists and dissidents. Most were educated, aligned themselves with the middle class and the professions, and were committed to assimilating into American society by learning and outwardly adopting American culture. In spite of their "Americanization," however, they maintained strong ties with the Polish community through the Polish church and community organizations. Although many foreign-born members of this group have developed excellent English skills, they not only speak Polish when amongst themselves, but also make sure their American-born offspring attend Polish church schools on weekends and develop a connection with the homeland through Polish dance, music, and even trips to Poland.

The third wave of immigrants began arriving in 1980. Although they may belong to either of the above groups economically, educationally, and socially, this third wave differs from the former two groups in that many came to the United States with the expectation that their move was temporary. Immigrants in this category often took any job that was offered and lived in low-income housing—often sharing with other immigrants. Many came on visitor's visas, leaving their families behind. Earnings were not spent to provide a better life in their new land, but were sent back to Poland. Health often suffered because of inadequate diets and the postponement of health treatment until a condition became severe. Although the current educational system in Poland is excellent and many were skilled laborers or even professionals in Poland, they often accepted unskilled positions for low wages. Because their visitor's visa did not allow them to work, they relied upon other Poles for sources of employment. In this group, there is no incentive to learn English or American culture because of the belief that their American sojourn will end soon and because they live entirely within Polish communities (often referred to as "Polonia") in northeastern and midwestern cities. Assimilation in these communities is slow because strong Polish religious and social organizations have provided schools, banks, and businesses as well as organizations dedicated to shipping goods and money to relatives in Poland.

Not all recent immigrants belong to this group. Many are well-educated professionals and businesspersons who bring their families along because they have made a conscious decision to resettle in the United States. They avoid Polonia because they feel uncomfortable there. These communities do not resemble the Poland they left behind. One commented that those he encountered in the largest Polonia in the United States, in Chicago, resembled, in speech and in dress, rural Poles of the era prior to World War II. While this third group of educated Poles work hard to assimilate American ways and culture, they often maintain a strong sense of pride in their Polish heritage. In contrast to Poles of the second wave of immigration who frequently shortened their names to "Americanize" them, members of the third wave rarely change their names.

Diversity in the Polish population. It is important for caregivers to understand this diversity in the Polish population when interacting with patients of Polish descent. Patient expectations for interaction with the physician and the healthcare institution will be strongly influenced by their attachments and relationship with the Polish community in the United States. Lack of fluency in English will not necessarily indicate how long the patient has been in the United States. Conversely, because the patient is a second generation Polish American and speaks English without an accent, the caregiver must not assume that that patient is fully in tune with mainstream American communication styles or health beliefs and practices.

Forms of Address

Most second and third wave Polish immigrants will expect caregivers to address all adults by Mr., Mrs., or Miss, followed by their family name. Although Polish names are often difficult for caregivers to pronounce, a Pole will value an attempt to pronounce his or her name correctly and any efforts made to learn the correct pronunciation. Although they may have difficulty in pronouncing the caregiver's family name, Polish patients will probably feel embarrassed if asked to address a caregiver by his or her first name.

One way of showing respect to someone whom one knows well but who is considered to be in a higher social position (possibly only due to age) is by placing the Polish equivalent of Mr., Mrs., or Miss before the person's first name or his or her title. A female physician, for example, might be addressed as *Pani Doctor* or "Lady Doctor" and a male physician as *Panie* (pronounced "Pan-yea") *Doctor* or "Mr. Doctor." The difference in these terms stems from the fact that the Polish language has gender and "cases" (i.e., a word takes a different ending according to its use in the sentence).

Other differences between the Polish and English languages that might affect a Pole's interaction with American caregivers are as follows:

In Polish it is considered rude to address someone with the second person *you*. Instead, Poles may substitute the person's name. Therefore, instead of asking, "Would *you* like me to sit over there?" the question might be phrased, "Would *the doctor* like me to sit over there?"

Polish is a language without articles (because the declension of words according to their function in a sentence renders articles unnecessary). As a result, nonnative English-speaking Poles often omit or misuse the words "the" and "a" when speaking English.

Attitudes and Behavior toward Physicians

Physicians hold an extremely high position in Polish society, although their pay is extremely low. The physician is considered an authority figure and, in general, patients will follow medical orders carefully. It is very uncommon for the patient to ask for a second opinion. This would be considered highly disrespectful to the physician. When patients do not fully trust the physician or feel that they are not getting better, they often change physicians. As in Russia and Bosnia, age and seniority are equated with knowledge, and patients in Poland often try to get their physician to send them to see "a professor." Because of the cultural attitude connecting age and wisdom, Polish American patients may be very distrustful of young residents and physicians.

Physicians are paid very poorly in Poland. For example, a third-year resident at a respected university hospital was paid the equivalent of $20 per month in 1986. Though pay has increased considerably since the collapse of communism, all but the top specialists are paid so poorly that they are forced to live at only a subsistence level. It is therefore common practice for patients and their families to present the physician with gifts in the form of goods or money to encourage extra attention or to thank him or her for quality care. American physicians should not feel insulted if an immigrant patient brings him or her a gift. Instead, it is important to explain that no gifts are necessary. If the gift is a small one (such as food or a souvenir of Poland) it might be graciously accepted. More valuable gifts will, of course, need to be returned with a polite explanation that physicians are not permitted to receive gifts from patients.

Patient Information Regarding Illness and Patient Involvement in Medical Decisions

Like many other cultural groups, Poles do not necessarily want a detailed knowledge of their illness or to participate in the choice of treatment. In Poland, it is common for laypeople to talk of having a "weak heart," a "bad liver," and so on. Friends and relatives will not question them about what kind of heart disease they suffer from or what kind of treatment they have received because it is assumed that the person will not know. Polish immigrant patients are therefore extremely uneasy with the American medical practice of educating the patient in great detail about the exact nature and prognosis of his or her disease. This knowledge is considered the domain of the physician. The physician's responsibility is simply to do what is necessary to make the patient well.

In Poland, a negative prognosis is almost never shared with the patient. A diagnosis of cancer of any kind will be kept from the patient because it would be considered a death sentence. The physician would be expected to modify any form of bad news in a manner that would give the patient hope for full or partial recovery.

Family Structure and Values

Traditionally the father was head of the Polish family and only the church (priest) had greater authority. However, in third and fourth generation Polish American families, the authority of both parents is much more equal. Traditional family values and loyalty are very strong. For many Poles, marriage is considered an institution of respect and economic solidarity rather than a romantic bond. This belief has contributed to the fact that older second and third generation Polish Americans have the lowest divorce rates of any White ethnic group. The high value placed upon family solidarity makes divorce a truly last resort.

Traditionally, it is a woman's duty to respect and obey her husband and a husband's duty to be loyal, to be faithful, and to financially support his wife. Adult children are expected to support their parents emotionally and financially. Thus, most first generation immigrants would consider it a disgrace to place the elderly in a nursing home. In a study of the ability of elderly emigrés from former Soviet bloc countries to adjust to nursing homes, it was found that Polish Americans (most in this study's population were elderly Poles who had spent most of their lives in Polonia) had the greatest difficulty adjusting to the nursing home environment. They expressed the feeling of being abandoned by their children. If placement in a nursing home is advised, it is crucial for both staff and other residents of the home to speak Polish and for Polish religious rituals, customs, and food to be an integral part of the institution.

Food and Hospitality: A Way of Life!

Food (and drink) is a very important symbol of hospitality, and guests in a Polish household will be offered food and be expected to eat. Because Poland is heavily forested and has short summers and long, cold winters, fish (except for freshwater carp) is scarce and the main meat staples are wild game and pork, while the main vegetables are root vegetables such as celery root, carrots, beets, and turnips. The cold weather encourages the consumption of stews and soups. Fats are drawn into the liquids and the vegetables and meats are cooked until they lose their nutritional value. A diet common to many first wave and rural Polish immigrants consists of a breakfast of coffee, bread, cheese, sausage (cooked or hard), and eggs. There is often a midmorning break of tea or coffee and a sandwich. The main meal is traditionally in midafternoon, and usually includes soup, meat, potatoes, cooked vegetable, and a dessert. The lighter evening meal consists of cold cuts, such as dried sausage, smoked ham, tongue, and head sausage, eggs, cheese, tomato, cucumber, and bread. This style of eating is often continued— except for the fact that the less easily digested main meal has been switched to the evening to accommodate a difference in working hours—in the homes of immigrants as well as their children born in the United States. In cases of obesity, high blood pressure, and so forth, caregivers are advised to question Polish American patients about their diet and provide education regarding healthier but culturally acceptable alternatives.

Social Structure, Interaction, and Communication Styles

Coming from a country where restaurants were expensive and not very good, Poles are used to socializing in one another's homes. When visiting a home, Poles often acknowledge the hostess by bringing flowers or candy. In spite of the great respect given the hostess, she will probably not expect guests to assist her in the kitchen or with cleanup after meals.

Polish-born males of the upper and educated middle classes often appear "old fashioned" when compared to American men. Even those who were brought up under "Communist equality" may have been trained at home to bow and kiss a woman's hand in greeting if it is offered. (This can cause some confusion when the American woman holds out her hand for a handshake!) Men have also been taught that it is polite to hold out a woman's chair for her to be seated and to hold open a door for a woman or for another male who is older or of higher social stature. New arrivals are thus often caught off guard in interactions with American women, who may view this kind of treatment as demeaning rather than respectful.

In general, Polish culture is a "touch" culture. In greeting relatives and close friends, Poles kiss three times: once on each cheek and once again. Men, as well as women, are used to embracing one another. This type of touching is not viewed as a sign of homosexuality, a lifestyle that is still very unaccepted in Poland and amongst Polish communities in the United States.

In spite of their informality with close friends, Polish Americans tend to be formal with strangers and healthcare providers. Handshaking is considered polite and will be done at each meeting. Punctuality is considered a form of respect and there is also a strong code for the "proper amount of time" that should be allotted to a visit. Social visits often seem to end abruptly because a first-time visitor considers he or she has stayed the "socially correct" amount of time.

Pregnancy and Childbearing Beliefs and Practices

The high value placed upon family makes the bearing of children a very important element of family life. Although the Catholic Church forbids birth control and abortion, the primary method of birth control in Poland during the 1970s and 1980s was abortion. When other forms of birth control were used, the IUD was selected over oral methods because of a fear and distrust of the pill. Immigrants of childbearing age as well as the children of immigrants often share this distrust.

The pregnant Polish woman will pay a great deal of attention to prenatal care and will make every effort to eat well and get adequate rest to ensure a healthy baby. She will seek care in a prenatal clinic if she cannot afford private care and will be careful to comply with medical advice. However, because of the traditional belief that the pregnant woman is "eating for two" it is important for the caregiver to monitor carefully the woman's weight gain during pregnancy and provide patient education about the dangers of putting on excess weight.

A woman is expected to rest for several weeks after delivery. It is common for her to take only minimal responsibility for the care of the newborn child. During these weeks of recovery, it is common for her mother or mother-in-law to step in and devote herself full time to these duties. The working mother and/or her parents may be shocked at the short amount of maternity leave given to women in the United States. In Poland, women are legally entitled to 90 days' leave with partial pay.

Second and third generation Polish immigrant women will wish to breast-feed their babies. This is one area where the caregiver or caregiving institution should provide counseling and education about breast-feeding techniques.

Childbirth

Childbirth is considered the "woman's" affair, and the woman traditionally remained isolated from both her husband and immediate family while in the labor and delivery room. The woman was admitted with labor pains and came out of the labor and delivery room with a child in her arms. Because of this tradition, Polish American husbands may feel very uncomfortable with the American custom of encouraging the husband's involvement in the labor and delivery. He should not be judged cold and uncaring if he does not wish to be present or participate.

Treatment of Infertility

Most Polish immigrants will find it very embarrassing and difficult to discuss details of the marital relationship with a third party. In spite of the high anxiety level regarding the woman's ability to conceive, Polish American couples tend to take a more passive approach and wait longer before seeking medical assistance than couples of other cultural groups.

Attitudes toward Mental Health

Physical (or even supernatural) basis for illness will always be considered before a mental one. Even immigrants who suffered the trauma of World War II and openly attribute their illness to these experiences rarely seek help from a psychiatrist or mental health professional. They are more likely to seek the advice of family, friends, or their priest. An Australian study of first-time admissions to psychiatric institutions has reported that amongst Eastern European refugees, there was a higher rate of admission of recent immigrants compared to earlier immigrants and a higher rate of admission for women than for men. One reason given for mental difficulties faced by immigrant Polish patients is that those who remain in Polonia shop in Polish stores, use their children as intermediaries when forced to interact with the American environment, and thus develop fewer coping skills for life in a new land.

Fatalism and Acceptance

Poles often have a strong sense of stoicism as well as a sense that "this illness or trouble was meant for me." This often leads the person to postpone seeking treatment until daily function is impaired—sometimes too late for a cure.

Death and Dying

Poles have a strong sense of family and hold the belief that they should take care of an immediate family member who is dying. Although they are usually willing to accept hospice care that is provided in the home, they may reject care outside the home. It is common for friends and family to wish to stay by the bedside of the dying person. Other friends and family may show their concern by bringing food, caring for children, and assisting in other ways.

It is customary to hold a wake for one to three days. This is followed by a Mass and a religious burial. The dead continue to be honored on All Souls Day (November 1) when the family attends a Mass and makes special offerings to the church. Family members also tend their loved one's gravesite by planting or bringing flowers and keeping it free from weeds.

Traditional Health Beliefs and Practices

Although there is a long tradition of biomedicine in Poland, it coexists with religious and herbal healers and a strong belief in holistic medicine. A "healer" who states that he has been given the gift of healing by the "laying on of hands" often gains a large following. Even educated and sophisticated Poles may believe that elements such as the weather, underground water currents, and stress influence their health. Before laying the foundations for a house, a diviner may be hired to locate underground water currents. This is because some believe that illness may be caused if a person's bed is positioned so that it crosses, rather than is placed in the same direction as, an underground current. When asked what they think has caused their illness, some Poles may tell you that their problems are simply due to having had "a hard and difficult life."

Strong religious faith supports a belief in the supernatural healing powers of persons and sanctuaries. One of the most famous is the icon of the virgin in St. Mary's Church in Chestohowa, Poland. This icon is surrounded by crutches and other offerings that have been left by crippled pilgrims who supposedly walked away whole and healthy again.

An important indication that a Pole, especially an older person, may hold a strong belief in spiritual healing and supernatural powers is religious medals that might be pinned to the patient's undergarments. These should not be removed or ridiculed, but should suggest careful questioning regarding the patient's view of the cause of the illness and what he or she has been doing or taking to treat the problem.

Natural/Holistic Cures

In Poland, holistic medicine is much more accepted than it is in the United States. Physicians often prescribe herbal medications that are filled at pharmacies. Tincture of valerian is often prescribed as a sedative and tincture of belladonna for peptic ulcer. Herbal teas such as *hyperci* are used for indigestion. Dill tea, for example, is used for colic and gas pains in newborns and infants. Chamomile tea is prescribed for upset stomach and externally as a disinfectant and for vaginitis. Many Polish immigrants have continued to grow herbs for medicinal purposes after coming to the United States. The popularity of this tradition is discussed in such publications as *Polish Herbs, Flowers & Folk Medicine* by Sophie Hodorowicz Knab (see Appendix C).

Polish immigrants often have a great trust in "natural" medications and may use them in addition to what the American caregiver prescribes. In order to avoid "double-dosing" with a combination of natural and manufactured medications, it is essential that caregivers carefully question patients regarding use of herbal or other forms of medications.

Health Problems and Concerns Common to Members of Polish Culture

1. *Heart disease, respiratory diseases, and obesity* (particularly in women) are some of the most common health problems of new immigrants. A lifestyle in Poland that did not include physical exercise as a common leisure-time activity, a high incidence of smoking, and a high-fat, high-cholesterol diet are contributing factors in these diseases.
2. *Respiratory disease and cancer as a result of pollution and radiation.* Many Polish immigrants living in Polonia communities worked or lived in close proximity to factories and steel plants in Poland that were built after World War II. These were constructed without filtering systems and were located close to major cities. Hence, a large percentage of this population was exposed to excessive pollution, thereby contributing to a high incidence of respiratory disease and cancer. Immigrants from Eastern Poland arriving after the Chernobyl incident in Russia may also have been exposed to radiation filtration into land and water systems.
3. *Tuberculosis, infant mortality, psychoneurosis, cardiovascular disease, musculoskeletal disorders, and alcoholism* were the major Polish health problems of the 1970s.
4. *Tooth decay* may also be a problem because of a shortage of dentists in Poland.

Suggested Screening

Polish immigrants should be screened for cardiac diseases, alcoholism, respiratory conditions, thyroid disorders (Poland stopped using iodized salt throughout the 1980s), and cancer—particularly leukemia.

Suggestions for Caregivers of Polish Americans

1. *Try to ascertain to which wave of immigrants the patient belongs and whether the patient lives within a Polonia or as part of a diverse American community.* The history of the patient and the patient's family will influence health beliefs and practices as well as patient/caregiver interaction.

2. *Address patients by their last name,* do not expect them to use your first name, and shake hands.

3. *Question the patient indirectly to learn whether or not the patient has consulted someone else* about his or her illness and whether this person was another family member or healer.

DEVELOPING CULTURAL PERSPECTIVE

1. What cultural factors might predispose a Polish American to heart disease and obesity?

2. Do Soviet Bloc émigrés trust the opinion of a nurse or a medical assistant? Why or why not?

3. An émigré might object to a routine diagnostic procedure yet be willing to be admitted into the hospital for a minor illness. Why?

4. How are mental health issues viewed by Bosnians?

5. Polish Americans equate age with wisdom. What would you do to instill the patient's confidence in a young but very skilled physician?

6. What sources of frustration would a Bosnian patient encounter within the Western medical establishment?

BLENDING PERSPECTIVES

1. Soviet Bloc countries have not had the same environmental safeguards as the USA. As a result, patients may have been breathing higher levels of pollutants. Should routine chest X-rays be recommended for patients from the Soviet Bloc?

2. Many émigrés are used to diets high in chicken fat, other fats, and starch. Can you think of ways to "ease" them into new eating habits? Do you have your "comfort foods" that are not healthy? What have you done to change your eating habits?

Chapter 8

The Effect of Religious Beliefs on Healthcare

Religious values and beliefs can have a strong effect on an individual's healthcare decisions and his or her compliance with a treatment plan. It is helpful, therefore, for caregivers to acquire a basic knowledge of the main tenets of their patients' religious beliefs and practices. Understanding and respecting religious teachings regarding lifestyle, reproductive practices, birth, and death, as well as religious restrictions concerning food, alcohol, caffeine, and other substances, will have a significant effect not only on the relationship between the caregiver and the patient but also on the patient's adherence to medical interventions, treatment plans, and recommended lifestyle changes.

Avoiding Stereotypes

It is essential for the caregiver not to assume that because a given patient is a member of a particular religious sect or group, he or she adheres to all or even some of the teachings of that religion. Knowledge about the religious beliefs of individual patients can be gained through a patient interview, as discussed in the introduction, and by asking the patient questions based on the set of tips at the end of this chapter. In this way, the caregiver can determine a patient's religious/spiritual beliefs and how these beliefs might affect lifestyle, treatment, and methods of health maintenance.

Organization and Contents

The religious beliefs summarized in this chapter are limited to those that have not been discussed earlier in this book.

The importance of religious beliefs on lifestyle and healthcare is frequently ignored. This chapter summarizes some aspects of religious belief and practice that might explain a patient's lifestyle or his or her failure to comply with a treatment plan, or that might affect the patient's (or the family's) decision-making process. The intent of this chapter is to broaden the caregiver's perspective on the interdependency of religion and health, and to increase sensitivity to the diverse needs of patients.

AMISH (OLD ORDER AMISH)

The Amish are a branch of the Mennonites,* direct descendants of Swiss Anabaptists who emigrated to the United States in the early 1700s to escape religious persecution. The Amish practice strict separation from the world by living in closed communities, and they speak a form of German as their first language. Although Lancaster County, Pennsylvania, is home to the oldest Amish settlement, which now numbers about 18,000 Amish, Amish communities can be found in twenty-one states as well as in Canada and South America. The Amish lifestyle has changed little from its sixteenth-century origins, and Amish still follow a strict religious life and avoid use of any modern technology. The Amish refer to outsiders as "English" and keep their distance from them, preferring to take care of their own. Visits to a clinic or practitioner are usually made only in an emergency or after family and community remedies have failed.

Aging parents usually live with children, and life and leisure time center around family, church, and community. Since children are only educated through the eighth grade or age sixteen (the minimum requirement set by the federal government), the Amish community does not produce its own physicians or nurses. Thus the Amish remain dependent on the "English" for all healthcare that goes beyond home remedies and natural cures.

The making and keeping of medical appointments is very difficult because the Amish are prohibited from owning automobiles (although not from riding in them) and reject worldly devices such as telephones. Televisions, central heating, air conditioning, refrigerators, and indoor toilets are very rare in an Amish community. The usual form of transportation is horse and buggy.

Another deterrent to receiving healthcare by licensed physicians and nurses is cost. In general, the Amish are an agrarian community. With the decreased availability of farmland, some Amish men have adopted other occupations such as carpentry, masonry, blacksmithing, or even industrial work in nearby factories. Women are usually homemakers. They and their children help out with farming chores and tend a home vegetable garden. The Amish are exempt from paying social security and Medicare payroll taxes and few, if any, receive any social security or other government benefits. They rarely have any kind of health or life insurance. Medical expenses, when incurred, are the responsibility of the family, with the help of a community fund contributed to by all of the families.

The Amish View of Health and Illness

Because the Amish define a "well" person as someone who has a good appetite, looks physically well, and can put in a good day's work, the Amish often postpone any form of treatment until the symptoms are so severe that the person can no longer work. In the case of a child's illness, it is the father rather than the mother who decides whether or when medical treatment should be sought.

Folk Medicine

The few existing studies of health practices in the Amish community report a strong tradition of family care for the sick and elderly. This care is largely dependent upon natural treatments such as vitamins and health foods, as well as

---

*Mennonites today are distinguishable enough from Amish also to be referred to as "English." Although Mennonite women dress in a manner similar to that of the Amish, men are sometimes clean-shaven and often wear modern-style clothes. Faithful Mennonites believe that the only life that is acceptable to God is lived in obedience to the Holy Scriptures. One Mennonite described the difference between the two groups in this way: "Whereas the Amish are opposed to anything that is modern, Mennonites are only opposed to that forbidden by the Scriptures." Mennonites do not forbid the use of electricity and are allowed to drive and own motorized vehicles.

folk remedies such as applying a poultice of smashed onion on the chest to help relieve congestion.

Although the Amish do not like to take even such over-the-counter drugs as aspirin, they are free to take vitamins and food supplements that are considered "natural" and, therefore, safe. Amish newspapers often carry advertisements for folk remedies and patent medicines. Many home gardens have a special place reserved for medicinal plants and herbs.

Some Amish still practice a form of folk medicine called *brauche,* or *powwowing,* a kind of physical manipulation in which the person with the gift of healing draws the illness from the body by placing his or her hands near the head or abdomen. This old-world form of faith healing uses words, charms, and amulets along with the physical manipulation. Perhaps this is why both chiropractors and reflexologists are usually readily accepted as appropriate healers.

Fertility, Birth, and Death

Birth control and abortion are forbidden, although a small number of Amish women are reported to use birth control. The average number of live births per family is seven. Each child is welcomed as a gift from God and a pregnancy is never terminated, even to save the woman's life. Because of the high fertility rate and the fact that the number of people who leave the church is small, the Amish population is increasing. Birth is usually a family and community responsibility and every effort is made to avoid "English" healthcare institutions. In fact, one study showed that out of 472 Amish pregnancies in Pennsylvania, while 90 percent of first births were performed in a hospital, only 59 percent of last births were performed outside of the home. Almost one-fourth of the women did not seek prenatal care until the sixth month of pregnancy.

Because of strong family ties, the sick and dying are almost always cared for at home.

Death is considered part of the natural rhythm of life and the dead are believed to have an eternal life with God.

Immunizations

Although most states require children to have immunizations before starting school, many Amish families present waivers on religious grounds. A survey of 100 Amish families showed that only 26 percent of children had been immunized against diphtheria, pertussis, and tetanus; 23 percent against poliomyelitis; and 16 percent against mumps and measles.

Health Risks

A health survey that involved asking 400 Amish to self-report their health in regard to hypertension, obesity, and stress indicated that hypertension was lower among Amish than non-Amish men and women. Self-reports of obesity were higher in Amish women than in Amish men, as were stress and depression. Amish women were significantly more likely to indicate that they felt depressed or low and that they felt stress strongly enough so that it interfered with their daily activities.

Caring for the Amish

Nurses and nurse practitioners working in Amish communities recommend flexibility and modification of standard practices and policies to accommodate Amish lifestyle and beliefs. Caregivers need to be aware that the Amish will only accept treatments that they feel are appropriate and will not hesitate to discontinue treatments they consider inappropriate and seek care elsewhere. The eighth-grade educational level of most Amish should be taken into consideration when advising patients and giving medical instructions. Caregivers working in Amish communities recommend such things as learning to rely more heavily on one's own clinical skills and judgment to avoid unnecessary tests. Because of the Amish distrust for the "English," caregivers also stress the need to participate actively, both professionally and as a citizen, in community activities such as selling quilts and church picnics. One nurse even reported trying Amish home remedies on herself and her daughter.

CHRISTIAN SCIENTISTS

The First Church of Christ, Scientist was established in Boston, Massachusetts, in 1879. A Bible-based system of spiritual healing, the Christian Science religion was founded by Mary Baker Eddy, who experienced personal healing in 1866 after having read an account of healing by Jesus in the New Testament. In 1875, Eddy published *Science and Health with Key to the Scriptures* and spent more than four decades teaching others how to heal and personally communicating a message of hope, healing, comfort, and strength through the Bible. In 1908, Eddy founded the *Christian Science Monitor*, a newspaper that is internationally known. There are now more than two thousand branches of the Church of Christ, Scientist in about eighty countries.

Christian Scientists believe that healing comes through God's response to prayer and make a conscious choice of prayer over medicine. The purpose of prayer is to heal by establishing harmony in all aspects of life. When one is healed there is both a moral and spiritual change.

There is little in the medical literature about caring for Christian Scientists. There have been, however, a number of well-publicized court cases against Christian Science parents who have withheld care from seriously ill children. Christian Scientists are not forbidden to use physicians. However, they often avoid diagnostic tests and will not accept any medical treatment that they believe is in violation of their religious beliefs, such as surgical procedures or medications. Christian Scientists believe that no disease is beyond the power of God to heal.

Fertility, Birth, and Death

The use of fertility drugs and artificial insemination is unusual, but birth control is left as an individual decision. Physicians or midwives are usually involved in births. Euthanasia is not permitted, nor are efforts to extend life usually supported.

Dietary Restrictions

There are no dietary restrictions for Christian Scientists, although alcohol and tobacco are forbidden and some Christian Scientists may also abstain from tea and coffee.

Transfusion and Organ Donation

The use of blood and blood products is not usually accepted as a medical treatment. Although organ donation is not forbidden, it is unlikely that a Christian Scientist will either search for or become an organ donor.

Caring for Christian Scientists

Caregivers should clarify whether and to what extent the patient and his or her family wish to abstain from medical and psychological procedures and medications and try to comply with these wishes. Care should be taken to learn the wishes of the patient or parent in life-threatening situations.

EASTERN ORTHODOX CHRISTIANS

The Eastern Orthodox Church encompasses many branches, such as the Greek, Ukrainian, Russian, and Rumanian Orthodox Churches. They each share the belief that they are the true reflection of Jesus and His Apostles, and do not believe in the authority of the Western Catholic Pope. Most Eastern Orthodox Christians follow the Orthodox Old Calendar, or Julian calendar, while some, such as the Greek and Cypriot Orthodox Churches, follow the Orthodox New Calendar, in which the Gregorian calendar is used for fixed holidays such as Christmas, and the Julian calendar is used for calculating Easter and all related moveable feasts.

Although the Russian and Rumanian branches of the Orthodox Church have the largest number of adherents worldwide, the Greek Orthodox Church is the largest in both Europe and North America. The term "Greek Orthodox" has become more widely used than "Eastern Orthodox" to refer to those who follow the teachings of the Orthodox Church in these regions.

About 1.2 million people of Greek ancestry live in the United States, and many followers of other forms of Orthodox Christianity also attend Greek Orthodox Churches. The majority of Greeks live in New York and Chicago. Greek communities center around the church. The emphasis is upon faith rather than Bible readings or specific tenets. Many Greek Americans consider themselves religious even if they only attend church for the major holidays, baptisms, and funerals. The most important holy day is Easter and most Greeks attend church on that day.

Faith is considered an important factor in both maintaining and regaining health. Prayers may be offered to specific saints who may be asked to act on behalf of someone who is ill. Greeks tend to hold a strong belief in miracles, even if they are third-generation Americans. Icons are extremely important, and many Greeks display icons in their homes or offer candles to icons of specific saints at church. When a person is ill, the icon of the family saint or the saint for which the person has been named may be placed over the bed.

The Mediterranean Diet

There is little in the medical literature about the effect of the Eastern Orthodox tradition on health beliefs, practices, and care. However, in light of the recent interest in what is being called the "Mediterranean Diet," there have been a number of studies of the traditional diets of Greece. Greeks who follow the Greek Orthodox Church's requirements regarding fasting have been shown to have a significantly lower level of LDL/HDL than those who did not fast, after the results were adjusted for age, sex, BMI, and smoking.

Traditional Orthodox Christian custom involves a total of 180–200 days of fasting per year. The faithful avoid olive oil, meat, fish, milk, and dairy products on all Wednesdays and Fridays, as well as follow three principal fasting periods during the year. In the 40 days before Christmas, meat, dairy products, and eggs are not allowed (in addition to the regular prohibitions for Wednesdays and Fridays). During Lent (the 48 days before Easter), fish and olive oil are only allowed twice a week while meat, dairy products, and eggs are forbidden. For the 15 days in August preceding Assumption, the same fasting rules apply as for Lent, except that fish is only allowed on August 6. Seafood such as shrimp, squid, cuttlefish, octopus, lobster, and crab, as well as snails, is allowed on fasting days.

Folk Beliefs and Practices

Many Greeks hold a strong belief in *matiasma*, or the evil eye. Those who saw the movie *My Big Fat Greek Wedding* may have noticed that people seemed to spit at a baby in its mother's arms. Spitting is supposed to ward off the evil eye, as is a small "eye" amulet often attached to children's clothing. When it is determined that an adult or child has been given the evil eye, ritual prayers may be said by family members or, in severe cases, by the Orthodox priest who may say prayers of exorcism and wave incense over the head and body of an afflicted person. Often herbal and tea remedies are tried as a self-treatment before visiting a physician. Because in Greece most drugs that require a prescription in the United States are readily available in pharmacies, Greeks may bring medications with them or ask relatives to send medications to them. Therefore, it is important to ask the patient what specific medications he or she is currently using or has used in the past.

Transfusion and Organ Donation

Some religious Greeks may not accept organ donation or readily consent to autopsy because of a belief in the physical resurrection of the body, but there are no restrictions on blood transfusion.

Caring for Orthodox Patients

Some Greeks distrust health professionals who are not also family members and may postpone visits to physicians for as long as possible. They may also shop around until they find a physician whom they feel is sympathetic and who offers a diagnosis and treatment plan that is acceptable. When a Greek is hospitalized, an icon, rather than a Bible, may be placed at the bedside. Most Greek immigrants view Americans as very formal and impersonal. They will respond more positively to caregivers who are friendly, ask about family, and show caring through touch.

JEHOVAH'S WITNESSES

This sect of Christianity was founded in Pennsylvania by Charles Taze Russell in 1872 and now numbers over six million members worldwide. The name was taken from the Hebrew-Christian faith, where Jehovah is Judge, Statute-giver, and King. The religious belief system of Jehovah's Witnesses is based upon a literal interpretation of the Bible. Accordingly, followers believe that humans are the result of divine creation and that human life, created by God, is sacred from the moment of conception. Man was created to live forever and physical death is only temporary for those who have been reborn by accepting Jesus Christ as Savior and following His teachings. On Judgment Day, believers will be resurrected to eternal life.

Transfusion and Organ Donation

Because of their literal interpretation of the Old and New Testaments and the references in Genesis and Leviticus prohibiting the eating of the blood of life, Jehovah's Witnesses believe that blood transfusions are sinful and may cause the receiver of the blood to be excommunicated and to exist in a state of eternal damnation.

While there is precise doctrine regarding the acceptance of blood and blood products, there is no ruling on the donation or receipt of organs. The *Watchtower*, the official publication of the Jehovah's Witness sect, states that "[w]hile the Bible specifically forbids consuming blood, there is no Biblical command pointedly forbidding the taking in of other human tissue. Therefore, the decision to donate or receive an organ is left to individual choice as long as the transplantation process does not involve the use of blood or blood products."

Acceptable and Unacceptable Medical Procedures

While all Jehovah's Witnesses refuse homologous blood and its main fractions—plasma, red blood cells, white blood cells, and platelets, and preoperative storage of autologous blood for later use during surgery—there are a number of procedures that are acceptable to many, but not all, Jehovah's Witnesses. Some of these include normovolemic hemodilution, which involves the preoperative removal of a volume of blood from the patient with the simultaneous administration of crystalloid or colloid to maintain circulating volume; preoperative and postoperative blood salvage, which involves the removal by suction of blood from the operative field followed by washing, filtering, and return of red cells to the patient; use of products derived from the main components of blood (albumin, clotting factors, antithrombin III, synthetic hemoglobin); autotransplantation of stem cells; and transplant of solid organs. All Witnesses accept plasma substitutes not derived from blood, such as perfluorocarbons, erythropoietin, and hematopoietic agents obtained from genetic recombination. EPO (erythropoiesis with recombinant erythropoietin) is acceptable to Jehovah's Witnesses and has been used to facilitate high doses of chemotherapy with stem cell transplantation, pancreatic surgery, and in the management of acute upper gastrointestinal hemorrhage.

One study suggests that the simplest way to avoid using blood components and products is to limit blood loss from the patient. While limiting blood loss is not always possible, there are pharmacological agents available to reduce blood loss in the surgical setting.

Ethical and Legal Considerations

Many caregivers are uncomfortable accepting Jehovah's Witnesses as patients, especially for surgical procedures (including obstetrics) and in oncology where chemotherapy often results in anemia. However, despite the conflict between the caregiver's medical pledge to do no harm and the patient's constitutional right to refuse treatment, the refusal of Jehovah's Witnesses to receive transfusions has resulted in many medical advances that avoid the use of blood and blood products.

When a mentally competent adult declines medical treatment, a court will not overrule this decision. If the patient is unconscious, and no other information is available, a transfusion should be administered if indicated. Should a family member refuse a transfusion for an unconscious patient whose wishes are not known, an emergency court order should be sought. In the case of children of Jehovah's Witnesses, the decision depends on the age of the child. The Family Reform Act of 1969 allows children over 16 years of age to make their own decisions, but in any case, legal advice should be sought from an expert in medical law. In an emergency, a lifesaving transfusion may be administered to a minor without parental consent, but it is recommended that two senior physicians document the circumstances and need for this procedure.

Caring for a Jehovah's Witness Patient

It is paramount to recognize the fact that not all Jehovah's Witnesses adhere to the same beliefs and some may agree to accept blood or blood products in emergency circumstances. It is important that physicians question each patient in private about these issues so as to avoid undue influence of others. It is also important that the physician make a personal decision regarding whether he or she is willing to let a patient die because of his or her beliefs before accepting care of that patient. If not, and the patient is adamant about refusal of a possibly lifesaving blood transfusion, the physician should assist in placing the patient in the care of another physician who would be willing to accept the consequences of the patient's decision.

Most Jehovah's Witnesses present a healthcare proxy that clearly outlines what interventions are acceptable. This signed document, renewed yearly, requests that their position on the refusal of blood be respected even when their life is at risk. The Division of Maternal-Fetal Medicine of the Department of Obstetrics, Gynecology and Reproductive Science at Mount Sinai Medical Center in New York has developed specific forms and protocol for treating Jehovah's Witness obstetrical patients. (See Gyamfi et al., Appendix C, for the report that includes these forms and protocol. This report also suggests the discussion of end-of-life decisions and assigning next of kin to children.)

JEWS

There are about 5.3 million Jewish people in the United States today. They may be affiliated with the Orthodox, Conservative, or Reform streams of Jewish practice, depending upon their adherence to Jewish laws and practices as reflected in the Torah (the five books of Moses that are the basis of the Jewish faith), the Talmud (commentaries on the Torah), or traditions that have developed over time. Other Jews remain unaffiliated with any formal religious branch.

Matrilineal Descent

In Orthodox and Conservative Judaism, any child of a Jewish mother is considered Jewish, even if the mother has converted to another religion. In the case of donor eggs, the heritage of the gestational mother, rather than that of the donor mother, determines the religion of the child. When a woman converts to Judaism during pregnancy, the child will be considered Jewish. If she converts after the child is born, that child would have to undergo conversion to Judaism. Reform Judaism's rules and traditions are less strict. If either parent is Jewish, the child is considered Jewish. Reflecting these differences in traditions, a child born of a Jewish father and a non-Jewish mother is Jewish by Reform tradition, but not by Conservative or Orthodox tradition.

Dietary Laws and Restrictions

Jewish dietary laws, or *kashrut* (kosher), are strictly followed by all Orthodox Jews, but rarely by Reform Jews. Conservative Jews vary in how strictly they follow the rules of *kashrut*. Keeping kosher requires that all food be prepared in a kitchen that is kosher and served on dishes that are kosher.

To be kosher, meat must come from an animal that has cloven hooves and chews its cud. Beef, lamb, and chicken can be kosher if killed according to Jewish law, but pork cannot. A special butcher called a *schochet* must slaughter the animal in a prescribed fashion. The meat must be *kashered* (soaked and salted) to remove blood and only certain parts of the meat can be eaten. There are rules governing fish, too. Fish must have fins and scales in order to be kosher. This means that shellfish such as shrimp, lobster, scallops, or clams are forbidden. Because of the strict regulations regarding the slaughtering and preparation of meat, many Orthodox Jews will not eat meat unless prepared by someone they know personally and may also refrain from eating fish in restaurants that are not kosher.

Kosher Jews do not eat or drink milk or dairy products at the same time as they eat meat. The amount of time they must wait between dairy and non-dairy consumption can vary from three to six hours. Separate sets of dishes and utensils are maintained for meat products and dairy foods, and neither can be eaten from a dish meant for the other.

It is important that caregivers understand the degree to which these rules are observed by patients. If kosher food is brought to the patient by family, it cannot be heated in institutional appliances or served on institutional dishes. Kosher Jewish patients will normally seek care in a hospital set up to serve kosher meals, but those who may find themselves in a non-kosher facility may order vegetarian meals to avoid such issues.

The Sabbath

Sabbath candles are lit at sundown on Friday nights. This ritual is performed by Jewish women. In hospitals and homes where oxygen is present, electric candles may be substituted.

Those who strictly observe the Sabbath will refrain from all forms of work on the Sabbath, which extends from sundown on Friday until after sundown on Saturday. Orthodox Jews will not turn on or off any electrical appliance during this period. This means that those in the hospital may be unwilling to use an electric call button, an elevator, an electric bed, or even a self-administered pain reliever.

Observant Jews may not carry money or identification on the Sabbath because carrying anything is considered work. Riding in automobiles, taxis, or buses is also prohibited, although in a medical emergency, this will be waived. As soon as the emergency has passed, however, the Sabbath rules take precedence and the Orthodox patient may refuse to be discharged until after the Sabbath. Also, the family of a deceased person may refuse to have the body moved until after the Sabbath.

Pregnancy and Birth

In the Orthodox practice of Judaism, having children is viewed as fulfilling God's commandment to be fruitful and multiply. Procreation is considered both an obligation and a blessing and contraception, therefore, is discouraged except when pregnancy might jeopardize the health of the mother. Although abortion is against Jewish law, it is not viewed as murder. Abortion may be permitted during the first 40 days after conception because the zygote is not yet viewed as a person. For the rest of the pregnancy, since the fetus is considered a part of the mother and one should not desecrate the human body, elective abortion is forbidden. Some Jews may avoid making preparations for a baby before it arrives because of a superstition that it may bring bad luck. They may shop for the new baby but not bring their purchases into the house before the baby is born safely.

The Orthodox husband may not wish to be present during delivery or remain as long as the woman's genital area is uncovered. The chief labor support may come from a woman from the family or community. Orthodox women traditionally wear a head covering or wig and if this needs to be removed, they should be provided with a surgical cap or other form of cover. If the husband's religious practice does not allow any form of physical contact with adult women, it would be inappropriate for a female physician or nurse to hand him the baby.

Male children are circumcised by ritual on the eighth day of life by a specially trained person called a *mohel*. This ritual is so important that it may even be performed on the Sabbath or on any holy day. However, many non-Orthodox Jewish parents choose to have their son circumcised in the hospital rather than at a formal *bris*. Therefore, it is important to clarify the wishes of the parents prior to birth. Boys are named during this ceremony whereas girls are usually named in the synagogue on the Sabbath after birth.

Prevalent Illnesses

Genetic conditions such as Tay-Sachs disease, Canavan disease, Fanconi anemia, Gaucher disease, cystic fibrosis, and some forms of genetically transmitted cancer may occur in the Ashkenazi Jewish population (descendants of central and eastern European Jews). Couples of this origin may seek genetic counseling or testing prior to marriage or before beginning a family. In Orthodox communities where marriages may be arranged, pre-engagement testing may be performed.

Organ Donation

While there is strong proscription against body mutilation, the saving of a life is even more important; therefore, organ donation is permitted as long as it does not involve the hastening of the death of another.

Death and Dying

The body is considered God's property and must be treated with respect. In general Jews do not believe in autopsies. However, most families will agree to one if (1) it is legally required; (2) three physicians certify that the cause of death cannot be determined without one; (3) three physicians certify that it might save the lives of others who suffer from the same illness; and (4) the findings of an autopsy might benefit surviving relatives in the case of a possible hereditary illness. Jewish law requires prompt burial—usually within 24 hours. Embalming or other means of preservation is not customary.

MORMONS (CHURCH OF JESUS CHRIST OF LATTER-DAY SAINTS)

The Church of Jesus Christ of Latter-day Saints (LDS) was founded in 1830. Its founder, Joseph Smith, believed that he was instructed by the angel Moroni to unearth a set of golden tablets containing God's last testament to the world. This testament became the Book of Mormon and its followers are most commonly called Mormons. However, most members of this religion refer to themselves as Latter-day Saints or members of the Church of Jesus Christ of Latter-day Saints, or LDS. There is also another, smaller group with Mormon roots, but with a much different belief system, called the Community of Christ, formerly known as the Reorganized Church of Jesus Christ of Latter-day Saints or the RLDS Church.

After Smith's death, Brigham Young led the LDS community west to escape religious persecution and finally established their religious center in Salt Lake City. There are now more than 12 million members worldwide and the church remains the fastest growing Christian denomination in the United States. This growth may be attributed to a strong commitment to converting others (all young men between the ages of 19 and 21 spend two years as missionaries and young women spend 18 months) and a birth rate that is the highest in the United States (see "Childbearing and Child Rearing," below).

General Health and Healthcare

About 70 percent of the population of the state of Utah belongs to the Church of Jesus Christ of Latter-day Saints, representing the highest concentration of any single religion in the United States. Utah also has the highest concentration of adults 18 years of age and over who are married with children living in the household. It has the lowest percentage of current smokers and binge and chronic drinkers. The LDS strongly support both education and world-class healthcare. Because life is considered sacred, religious prohibitions can be waived to comply with medical advice regarding the health and life of the patient.

Religious Beliefs and Practices

The primary scriptures of the LDS are the King James Version of the Bible, the Book of Mormon, the Doctrine and Covenants, and the Pearl of Great Price. Churches are the center of Sunday worship and weekly community activities, but major temples such as the Tabernacle are often used for marriages and special religious events. There are no professional clergy and each member of the LDS church has a church-designated home teacher who visits on a regular basis. The home teacher will visit the hospital patient, say prayers for his or her welfare, anoint the sick or offer the sacrament of the Lord's Supper (a form of communion). If a member of LDS is hospitalized away from home, he or she may ask a hospital chaplain to contact the local Mormon congregation to ask them to provide a member for spiritual support and care.

Sundays are set aside for worship, and Monday nights are designated as "family home evenings," a time when family members gather for religious instruction, prayer, and recreation.

Family Roles

Family life is the basic unit of the religion. The LDS family follows a patriarchal system in which the husband presides over the family and is the primary provider of the physical and spiritual needs of his wife and children. Women have a very prominent role in the LDS Church. They bear the children, manage the household, and actively contribute to the religious education of their children. Children are given family duties appropriate to their age and abilities, such as watching over younger siblings.

Childbearing and Child Rearing

Mormons believe strongly in the scriptural injunction to multiply and replenish the Earth. The family is viewed as an eternal entity and the bonds of marriage are considered sacred. Both premarital sex and adultery are prohibited as are birth control and abortion, unless the pregnancy places the woman's health at risk. Childbearing is considered one of the Mormon woman's most significant roles. She is believed to be creating a body for a child of God. Since the female body is regarded as the tabernacle of the spirit and the residence of a child of God, high priority is given to prenatal care. Most women see their physicians regularly and give birth in hospitals. In the postpartum period, routine household duties are performed by members of the family, church, or community so that the woman can rest. Breast-feeding is encouraged. A study of LDS women in Utah found that Mormon women had the lowest incidence of breast cancer in the United States and suggested that this low cancer rate was due to breast-feeding and multiple births. The study also reported that the average number of months of breast-feeding per child was greatest for those who attended church weekly.

Baptism

Baptism of children and converts is performed in church by full immersion. Children are not baptized until the age of eight—considered the age of accountability. Converts can be baptized at any age.

Dietary Restrictions

Mormons abstain from tobacco, alcohol, coffee, tea, caffeinated soft drinks, and illicit drugs. However, there is no ban on using medication containing alcohol or caffeine in cases where a healthcare professional deems it necessary to maintain or improve health.

Dress and Modesty

Faithful Mormons wear a religious undergarment, not unlike long underwear, with elbow-length sleeves and knee-length legs. This garment is not permitted to be exposed. It can be removed for sports, swimming, and for medical examinations in which a medical gown is needed. Should an LDS patient wish to wear this garment in the hospital setting, he or she should be allowed to wear pajamas from home to protect his or her modesty.

OTHER ASPECTS OF RELIGIOUS BELIEF AND MEDICAL CARE

Awareness of Religious Amulets and Symbols

Members of some religious groups may pin or sew amulets, beads, or other special symbols on their children to protect the wearer against the evil eye or evil spirits that they believe cause illness. If these items are removed by caregivers, even in preparation for surgery, the patient may fear a negative outcome of treatment.

Although most non-clerical Catholics in the United States do not wear rosaries, some Catholics from Italy and Mexico may wear them around their necks. In general, if a patient is wearing a rosary, permission must be gained before removing it. Permission may be more readily granted if the patient is allowed to hold the rosary in his or her hand or place it close to the bed or treatment table.

Some Southeast Asian patients may present for treatment wearing a string around their wrist or body indicating that they have probably visited a shaman about their illness prior to visiting the hospital or clinic. Single or multiple strings may have been tied to the wrists or body as a protection or cure. Because this symbol is believed to demonstrate spiritual wholeness and family support, it must be allowed to loosen or break by itself rather than be cut or removed on purpose. Whenever possible, it is best to sterilize the string or bracelet but leave it in place. When removal is necessary, it is important first to gain permission from the patient or the patient's family by explaining the reason for the request. Otherwise the patient may become depressed and refuse further treatment. Furthermore, he or she may blame the removal (and the person who removed it) for continued illness or the worsening of the patient's condition.

Hair in the Sikh Religion

Once male Sikh religious followers reach the age of maturity, they may not cut or shave any bodily hair. This rule has important implications for the procedures used in the cleansing of a wound or in preparing a patient for surgery. Even one of the common Sikh practices for keeping the male's beard tidy may create health hazards. This practice involves running a string from beneath the jaw around the ears and tying both ends together on top of the head, where it is hidden by the turban. As the beard grows, it is wrapped around the string, which gets tighter with each wrap. If the string becomes too tight, it may restrict the swallowing of big boluses of food and severely restrict the mouth opening and thus inhibit breathing. Since many Western caregivers are unaware of this practice, a simple diagnosis and treatment for the presenting symptoms of difficulty in swallowing and breathing in Sikh men often goes undiscovered.

These examples are presented to alert caregivers about the need to identify some of the beliefs and practices of the principal religious groups in their service area. These beliefs and practices may affect risk-management as well as the quality of healthcare. In order to develop trusting and beneficial relationships with members of various religious groups, institutions as well as individual caregivers must be willing to identify and understand their beliefs and practices, and modify care accordingly.

Tips for Offering Care to Diverse Religious Groups

1. Identify the patient's religious persuasion. Not all patients of a particular culture belong to the same religion nor do all members of the same religion practice the strictest dictates of that religion. Ask the patient or the patient's family whether there are any religious beliefs or restrictions that you need to be aware of as caregiver.

2. While examining the patient, try to note religious symbols, amulets, or other religious indicators. If the patient is wearing something that looks like a religious symbol, ask what it means and whether or not it may be removed if needed. Respect the patient's response and do not remove any religious object without first gaining the patient's (or the family's) permission to do so.

3. Ask patients whether or not they have consulted a member of their church or clergy or religious order for a health diagnosis or advice. If the patient has done so, ask what that religious advisor has given as the cause of the complaint and what was recommended as a cure. Do not be critical of other recommendations or methods of healing and try, if possible, to make your treatment plan seem to complement rather than contradict them.

4. Explain the treatment plan (but not necessarily the medical details of the treatment). Ask specifically whether there are any religious prohibitions to anything in the proposed treatment plan. If there are, work with the patient to modify the plan so that no religious precepts are breached.

5. Listen carefully to patient requests for a caregiver of the same sex. Try to determine whether this request is merely a preference or if there are any dictates of the patient's religion that require him or her to be examined by a member of the same sex. If there are religious requirements for same sex care, these should never be breached. Out of courtesy, try to comply with the patient's request in either case.

6. Be keenly aware of a parent's body language when you compliment the parent's infant or child. Remember that in some cultures a compliment must be accompanied by an appropriate gesture to avoid attracting the evil eye. If the parent seems upset or appears to counteract your compliment by saying something negative, either end your compliment or ask what gesture would be appropriate to accompany your remark.

7. In many Southeast Asian religions and cultures the head is thought to be the seat of life because the soul is believed to reside in the head. Always ask permission before touching the head of a patient. If it is necessary to perform any procedure involving the head, such as placing an intravenous line through an

infant's scalp, explain what will be done and why it is necessary before beginning the procedure.

8. Occasionally a patient or his or her relatives may ask permission to perform a religious ceremony in the clinic or in the patient's room. In most cases this will help the patient by providing religious support. Try to find out the nature of the ceremony and what will be done. Unless the ceremony will harm the patient, disturb other patients, or severely disrupt the institution's operations, the emotional strength provided will far outweigh any difficulties that might arise from allowing the ceremony to occur.

DEVELOPING CULTURAL PERSPECTIVE

1. Why should you be wary of praising infants and young children in front of their parents?

2. How could you maximize the success of your interactions with and treatments for an Old Order Amish patient?

3. How might standard hospital procedures be upsetting to:
   - a faithful Mormon
   - an Orthodox Jew
   - a Sikh

4. Why would an Old Order Amish patient delay medical treatment?

5. How do Christian Scientists view illness? What medical treatments will they accept?

BLENDING PERSPECTIVES

1. Some Jehovah's Witnesses reject blood transfusions, even if it means the death of a patient. What beliefs are you willing to die for? On the Sabbath some Orthodox Jews will not self-administer pain medication. What beliefs are you willing to suffer for?

2. In what verbal and nonverbal ways do you communicate your opinions of others' religious beliefs? How could you improve your style of interacting with patients and their families to foster their trust?

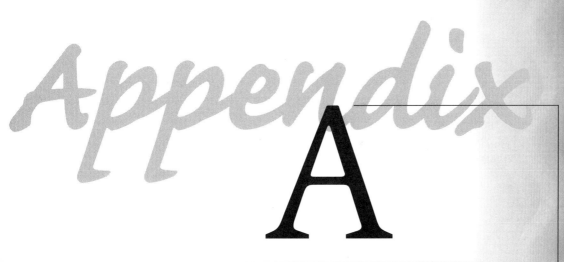

Discussion Questions on Cultural Perspective

1. Do you think cultural diversity training should be mandatory for all healthcare providers? Why or why not?

2. Does your healthcare facility have a "gift" policy? How might the policy be altered to accommodate belief systems about giving gifts to caregivers?

3. Some cultures value candor and some value an indirect approach. In which cultures would you modify a fatal prognosis by either giving the news in stages or avoiding the news altogether? What are the ethical implications of failure to provide the patient with the prognosis?

4. Provide examples of ways that cultural differences might affect how a patient views time and appointment promptness. How can a medical practice accommodate different perspectives of time?

5. How do cultural differences result in different expectations regarding the nature and quality of care as well as an understanding of what constitutes an appropriate patient/caregiver relationship? Provide specific examples.

6. The Greek humoral theory shows up in the belief system of many cultures. Do you think that the theory should be included in medical training? Why or why not?

7. Many cultures advocate self-treatment with herbs and folk remedies. Would standard medical history questions reveal use of these remedies? How would a clinician evaluate the safety of combining a particular remedy with a prescription medication? (Hint: Has standard pharmacological practice been amended to consider contraindications between common prescription medications and various herbs?)

8. Explain how the quality and availability of healthcare in other cultures alters patient advocacy. Is a patient who expects poor quality care as the norm more likely to be more aggressive in his approach and more insistent upon a second opinion? Will reciting the Patient's Bill of Rights to this patient alleviate his concerns or aggravate them?

9. Is it "right" or "fair" to let a child die because of his/her parents' religious convictions?

10. In what practical ways might you help your organization develop strategies aimed at increasing sensitivity to the needs of members of diverse religious groups who are in your care?

B

Guidelines for Communicating across Cultures

Tips for Successful Caregiver/Patient Interaction Across Cultures

1. Don't treat the patient in the same manner you would want to be treated.
2. Begin by being more formal with patients who were born in another culture.
3. Don't be "put off" if the patient fails to look you in the eye or ask questions about the treatment.
4. Don't make *any* assumptions regarding the patient's concepts about the ways to maintain health, the causes of illness, or the means to prevent or cure illness.
5. Allow the patient to be open and honest with you by not discounting or laughing at beliefs that are not held by our Western biomedical tradition.
6. Don't discount the possible effect of the belief in the supernatural on the patient's health and well-being.
7. Make your questioning indirect concerning the patient's belief in the supernatural or use of nontraditional forms of cure.
8. Try to ascertain the value of involving the entire family in the treatment.
9. Be cautious around issues of "informed consent."
10. Be very restrained in relating bad news or in explaining in detail the many complications that may result from a particular course of treatment.
11. Whenever possible, try to incorporate into your treatment plan the elements of the patient's folk medication and folk beliefs that are not specifically contraindicated.

Tips for Determining the Individual Etiquette, Beliefs, and Practices of Patients from Other Cultures

1. Introduce yourself formally, using title and last name, and ask the patient how he or she wishes to be addressed.
2. Ask the patient what he or she believes has caused the illness.
3. Ask the patient how they think the illness or complaint can best be cured.
4. Ask the patient if he or she has consulted anyone else about the complaint prior to coming to you.
5. Ask the patient how medical decisions are made in his or her culture.

6. Never assume that a patient will be familiar with a particular type of medical test or procedure.

7. Before prescribing a dietary regime, ask the patient what he or she usually eats, as well as how often and what time meals are eaten.

8. Be prepared to accept the fact that excellence in care will mean very different things to patients of different cultures.

Tips for Communicating Directly with Limited-English-Speaking Patients

1. Speak slowly, not loudly.
2. Face the patient and make extensive use of gestures, pictures, and facial expressions.
3. Avoid difficult and uncommon words and idiomatic expressions.
4. Don't "muddy the waters" with unnecessary words or information.
5. Organize what you say for easy access.
6. Rephrase and summarize often.
7. Don't ask questions that can be answered by "yes" or "no."
8. Check your understanding of the patient by paraphrasing what he or she has said.
9. Check the concept behind the word.
10. Don't burden the patient with decisions he or she is not prepared to make.

Tips for Improving the Effectiveness of Interpreters

1. Brief the interpreter
2. Explain information/ask questions in two or three different ways.
3. Avoid long or complicated sentences.
4. Keep it short.
5. Allow the interpreter "thought time."
6. Don't interrupt!
7. Don't be impatient!
8. Allow for the directness of English.
9. Utilize/read gestures and facial expressions.
10. Remember that "culture" may cause even a professional interpreter to modify what you or the patient has said.

Tips for Improving Patient Satisfaction and Compliance by Integrating Cultural or Folk Medical Practices and Beliefs into Your Treatment Plan

1. Learn about your patients' basic health/illness beliefs and practices by asking patients directly or indirectly about food and diet, medication, other forms of care, the body, and belief system.
2. Consider which of the above beliefs would not interfere with your plan of treatment or be contraindicated.
3. Avoid, whenever possible, a treatment plan that conflicts with the patient's beliefs and lifestyle.

Tips for Diet and Nutrition Assessment and Counseling

1. Learn something about the traditional diet and lifestyle of the cultures to which some of your patients belong.
2. Don't make any assumptions based on standard U.S. eating habits.
3. Identify the specific dietary changes undergone by immigrants since coming to the United States.
4. Try to identify taboos about particular foods.
5. Ask the person about beliefs in the special properties of certain foods.
6. When advising a patient that a change in dietary habits is necessary, try to negotiate changes that are healthful and appropriate.
7. Beware of the strong "pull" of a belief in fatalism in the unwillingness of some culturally diverse patients to change their diet and lifestyle.
8. There are biochemical reasons for some food choices or omissions in traditional diets.

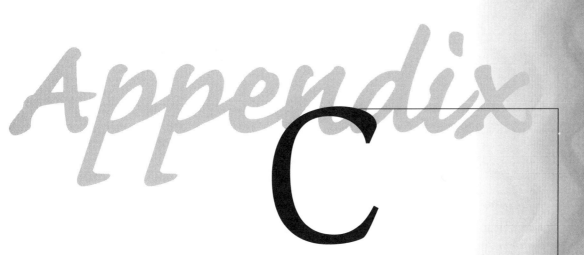

Sources for Further Reading

Chapter 2

Barrett, Ronald K. "Death and Dying in the Black Experience." *Journal of Palliative Medicine* 5, no. 5 (October 2002): 793–9.

Baskin, M. L., H. K. Ahluwalia, and K. Resnicow. "Obesity Intervention among African-American Children and Adolescents." *Pediatric Clinics of North America* 48, no. 4 (August 2001): 1027–39.

Braithwaite, Ronald L. and Sandra E. Taylor, eds. *Health Issues in the Black Community*. 2nd ed. San Francisco: Jossey-Bass, 2001.

Collins, Karen Scott, M.D., Katie Tenney, and Dora L. Hughes, M.D. *Quality of Health Care for African Americans: Findings from The Commonwealth Fund 2001 Health Care Quality Survey*. New York: The Commonwealth Fund, 2002. (This report is available upon request from *www.cmwf.org*.)

Jackson, Jacquelyne Johnson. "Urban Black Americans." In *Ethnicity and Medical Care*, edited by Allen Harwood. Boston: Harvard University Press, 1981.

Murphree, Alice. "A Functional Analysis of Southern Folk Beliefs Concerning Birth." *American Journal of Obstetrics and Gynecology* 102, no. 1 (1968): 125–34.

Russell, Kathleen, and Nancy Jewell. "Cultural Impact of Health-Care Access: Challenges for Improving the Health of African Americans." *Journal of Community Health Nursing* 9, no. 3 (1992): 161–9.

Snow, Loudell F. "Traditional Health Beliefs and Practices among Lower Class Black Americans." *Western Journal of Medicine* 139 (1983): 820–8.

_____. "Folk Medical Beliefs and Their Implications for Care of Patients: A Review Based on Studies among Black Americans." *Annals of Internal Medicine* 81 (1974): 82–96.

_____. "Sorcerers, Saints and Charlatans: Black Folk Healers in Urban America." *Culture, Medicine and Psychiatry* 2 (1978): 69–106.

Spector, Rachel E. *Cultural Diversity in Health and Illness*. 3rd ed. New Jersey: Appleton & Lange, 1991.

U.S. Department of Health and Human Services. "MentalHealth Care for African Americans." In *Mental Health: Culture, Race, and Ethnicity—A Supplement to Mental Health: A Report of the Surgeon General*. Rockville, MD: U.S. Department of Health and Human Services, Office of the Surgeon General, 2001.

Chapter 3

American Indian Health Service. "Heritage and Health" and "IHS Profile." *Health and Heritage Brochure*. http://info.ihs.gov.

Avery, Charlene. "Native American Medicine: Traditional Healing." *Journal of the American Medical Association* 265, no. 17 (1991): 2271–3.

Bell, Roxanne. "Prominence of Women in Navajo Healing Beliefs and Values." *Nursing & Health Care* 15, no. 5 (1994): 232–40.

Carrese, Joseph, and Lorna A. Rhodes. "Western Bioethics on the Navajo Reservation: Benefit or Harm?" *Journal of the American Medical Association* 274, no. 10 (1995): 826–9.

Dansie, Roberto. "Health from an Indian Perspective." *IHS Primary Care Provider* 22, no. 17 (1997): 116.

Hanley, Catherine E. "Navajo Indians." In *Transcultural Nursing*, 2nd ed., edited by Joice Newman and Ruth Elaine Davidhizar. St. Louis: Mosby, 1995.

Hatton, Diane C. "Health Perceptions among Older American Indians." *Western Journal of Nursing Research* 16, no. 4 (1994): 392–403.

Kunitz, Stephen, and Jerrold E. Levy. "Navajos." In *Ethnicity and Medical Care*, edited by Allen Harwood. Cambridge: Harvard University Press, 1981.

Locust, Carol, and Jerry Lang. "Walking in Two Worlds: Native Americans and the VR System." *American Rehabilitation* 22, no. 2 (1996): 2–14.

Schneider, Gregory W., and Mark J. DeHaven. "Revisiting the Navajo Way: Lessons for Contemporary Healing." *Perspectives in Biology and Medicine* 46, no. 3 (2003): 413–27.

Wilson, Kathleen. "Therapeutic Landscapes and First Nations Peoples: An Exploration of Culture, Health, and Place." *Health & Place* 9, no. 2 (2003): 83–93. *The IHS Primary Care Provider*, a journal for health professionals working with

American Indians and Alaska Natives, can be obtained free of charge from:

Department of Health and Human Services Indian Health Service Clinical Support Center Two Renaissance Square, Suite 780 40 North Central Avenue Phoenix, AZ 85004

Association of American Indian Physicians 1225 Sovereign Row, Suite 103 Oklahoma City, OK 73108

Chapter 4

General

Spector, Rachel E. "Health and Illness in the Asian-American Community." In *Cultural Diversity in Health and Illness.* 6th ed. Stamford, CT: Appleton & Lange, 2004.

Chinese

Chen-Louie, T. "Nursing Care of Chinese American Patients." In *Ethnic Nursing Care: A Multicultural Approach,* edited by M. S. Orque, B. Bloch, and L. S. A. Monrrowy. St. Louis: C. V. Mosby, 1983.

Kaptchuk, Ted. *The Web That Has No Weaver: Understanding Chinese Medicine.* New York: Congdon & Weed, 1983.

Kleinman, A. *Patients and Healers in the Context of Culture.* Berkeley: University of California Press, 1980.

Lai, Magdalene C., and Ka-Ming Kevin Yue. "The Chinese." In *Cross-Cultural Caring: A Handbook for Health Professionals in Western Canada,* edited by Waxler-Morison, J. M. Andersen, and E. Richardson. Vancouver: University of British Columbia Press, 1990.

Filipinos

Baysa, E., E. Cabrera, F. Camilon, and M. Torres. "The Pilipinos." In *Cross-Cultural Caring: A Handbook for Health Care Professionals in Hawaii,* edited by N. Palafox and A. Warren. Honolulu: University of Hawaii Press, 1980.

Cantos, A., and E. Rivera. "Filipinos." In *Culture and Nursing Care: A Pocket Guide,* edited by J. G. Lipson, S. L. Dibble, and P. A. Minarik. San Francisco: UCSF Nursing Press, 1996.

Hmong

Chan, Sucheng, ed. *Hmong Means Free: Life in Laos and America.* Philadelphia: Temple University Press, 1994.

Culhane-Pera, Kathleen A., Dorothy E. Vawter, Phua Xiong, Barbara Babbitt, and Mary M. Solberg, eds. *Healing by Heart: Clinical and Ethical Case Stories of Hmong Families and Western Providers.* Nashville: Vanderbilt University Press, 2003.

Fadiman, Anne. *The Spirit Catches You and You Fall Down: A Hmong Child, Her American Doctors, and the Collision of Two Cultures.* New York: The Noonday Press, 1997.

Jintrawet, Usanee, and Rosanne C. Harrigan. "Beliefs of Mothers in Asian Countries and among Hmong in the United States about the Causes, Treatments and Outcomes of Acute Illnesses: An Integrated Review of the Literature." *Issues in Comprehensive Pediatric Nursing* 26 (2003): 77–88.

South Asians

Fisher, J.A., M. Bowman, and T. Thomas. "Issues for South Asian Indian Patients Surrounding Sexuality, Fertility, and Childbirth in the US Health Care System." *Journal of the American Board of Family Practice* 16, vol. 2 (March/April 2003): 151–5.

Rajwani, Rozina. "South Asians." In *Culture and Nursing Care: A Pocket Guide,* edited by J. G. Lipson, S. L. Dibble, and P. A. Minarik. San Francisco: UCSF Nursing Press, 1996.

Chapter 5

Aguirre-Molina, Marilyn, Carlos W. Molina, Ruth Enid Zambrana, eds. *Health Issues in the Latino Community.* San Francisco: Jossey-Bass, 2001.

Caudle, Patricia. "Providing Culturally Sensitive Healthcare to Latino Clients." *Nurse Practitioner* 18, no. 12 (1993): 40, 43–6, 50–1.

Chisney, A., et al. "Mexican American Folk Medicine: Implications for the Family Physician." *Journal of Family Practice* 2, no. 4 (1980): 567–70.

Chong, Nilda. *The Latino Patient: A Cultural Guide for Health Care Providers.* Yarmouth: Intercultural Press, 2002.

Flores, Glenn. "Culture and the Patient-Physician Relationship: Achieving Cultural Competency in Health Care." *Journal of Pediatrics* 136, no. 1 (2000): 14–23.

Harwood, Alan. "The Hot-Cold Theory of Disease: Implications for Treatment of Puerto Rican Patients." *Journal of the American Medical Association* 216, no. 7 (1971): 1153–8.

Koss-Chioino, Joan D., and Jose M. Canive. "The Interaction of Popular and Clinical Diagnostic Labeling: The Case of *Embrujado.*" *Medical Anthropology* 15 (1993): 171–88.

Lagana, Kathleen. "Come Bien, Camina y No Se Preocupe—Eat Right, Walk, and Do Not Worry: Selective Biculturalism During Pregnancy in a Mexican American Community." *Journal of Transcultural Nursing* 14, no. 2 (2003): 117–24.

Logan, Michael H. "New Lines of Inquiry on the Illness of *Susto.*" *Medical Anthropology* 15 (1993): 189–200.

Maduro, Renaldo. "*Curanderismo* and Latino Views of Disease and Curing." *Western Journal of Medicine* 139 (December 1983): 868–74.

National Coalition of Hispanic Health and Human Services Organizations (COSSMHO). *Delivering Preventive Health Care to Hispanics: A Manual for Providers.* Washington, D.C., 1990.

Spector, Rachel E. "Health and Illness in the Latino-American Community." In *Cultural Diversity in Health and Illness.* 3rd ed. New Jersey: Appleton & Lange, 1991.

Chapter 6

General

Lipson, Juliene G., and Afaf I. Meleis. "Issues in Health Care of Middle Eastern Patients." *The Western Journal of Medicine* 139, no. 6 (December 1983): 854–61.

Salari, Sonia. "Invisible in Aging Research: Arab Americans, Middle Eastern Immigrants, and Muslims in the United States." *The Gerontologist* 42, no. 5 (October 2002): 580–8.

Shiloh, Ailon. "The Interaction between the Middle Eastern and Western Systems of Medicine." *Social Science & Medicine* 2, no. 3 (September 1968): 235–48.

Arabs

AbuGharbieh, Patricia. "Arab-Americans." In *Transcultural Health Care: A Culturally Competent Approach,* edited by Larry D. Purnell and Betty J. Paulanka. Philadelphia: F.A. Davis Company, 1998.

Laffrey, Shirley C., et al. "Assessing Arab-American Health Care Needs." *Social Science & Medicine* 29, no. 7 (1989): 877–83.

Meleis, Afaf Ibrahim. "Arab Americans." In *Culture & Nursing Care,* edited by Juliene G. Lipson et al. San Francisco: UCSF Nursing Press, 1996.

Meleis, Afaf Ibrahim, and Mahmoud Meleis. "Egyptian-Americans." In *Transcultural Health Care: A Culturally Competent Approach,* edited by Larry D. Purnell and Betty J. Paulanka. Philadelphia: F.A. Davis Company, 1998.

Meleis, Afaf Ibrahim, and Leila Sorrell. "Bridging Cultures: Arab American Women and Their Birth Experiences." *MCN, The American Journal of Maternal/Child Nursing* 6, no. 3 (May/June 1981): 171–6.

Zahr, Lina Kurdahi, and Marianne Hattar-Pollara. "Nursing Care of Arab Children: Consideration of Cultural Factors." *Journal of Pediatric Nursing* 13, no. 6 (December 1998): 349–55.

Iranians

Hafizi, Homeyra. "Iranians." In *Culture & Nursing Care,* edited by Juliene G. Lipson et al. San Francisco: UCSF Nursing Press, 1996.

Lipson, Juliene G. "The Health and Adjustment of Iranian Immigrants." *Western Journal of Nursing Research* 14, no. 1 (1992): 10–29.

Lipson, Juliene G., and Homeyra Hafizi. "Iranians." In *Transcultural Health Care: A Culturally Competent Approach,* edited by Larry D. Purnell and Betty J. Paulanka. Philadelphia: F.A. Davis Company, 1998.

Chapter 7
Bosnians

"Meeting the Needs of Bosnian Refugees." Written report of a meeting hosted by the Illinois Refugee Social Service Consortium and the Jewish Federation of Metropolitan Chicago, Feb. 27–Mar. 2, 1995.

Mollica, Richard F., M.D., et al. "Longitudinal Study of Psychiatric Symptoms, Disability, Mortality, and Emigration among Bosnian Refugees." *JAMA* 286, no. 5 (August 2001): 546–54.

Searight, H. Russell. "Bosnian Immigrants' Perceptions of the United States Health Care System: A Qualitative Interview Study." *Journal of Immigrant Health* 5, no. 2 (April 2003): 87–93.

Simic, Andrei. "Interpersonal Relationships among the South Slavs: Problems in Cross-Cultural Perception." *Serbian Studies,* published by the North American Society for Serbian Studies, 4, no. 4 (Fall 1988): 35–55.

Zander, Kathleen. *Bosnian Culture: A Profile in Minnesota.* The Center for Cross-Cultural Health: Minneapolis, 1997.

Poles

Aroian, Karen J. "Sources of Social Support and Conflict for Polish Immigrants." *Qualitative Health Research* 2, no. 2 (May 1992): 178–207.

Dunham, Daniel P., M.D., et al. "Dietary Differences among Women of Polish Descent by Country of Birth and Duration of Residency in the United States." *Ethnicity & Disease* 14, no. 2 (2004): 219–26.

From, Martha A. "People of Polish Heritage." In *Transcultural Health Care: A Culturally Competent Approach,* edited by Larry Purnell and Betty J. Paulanka. Philadelphia: F. A. Davis Company, 2003.

Hatchett, Richard. "Accepting the Challenge of the Past: Polish Medicine in the Period of Transition." *The Pharos* (Winter 1995): 34–8.

Knab, Sophie Hodorowicz. *Polish Herbs, Flowers & Folk Medicine.* New York: Hippocrene Books, 1995.

Wiking, Eivor, Sven-Erik Johansson, and Jan Sundquist. "Ethnicity, Acculturation, and Self Reported Health. A Population Based Study among Immigrants from Poland, Turkey, and Iran in Sweden." *Journal of Epidemiology and Community Health* 58 (2004): 574–82.

Russians

Aroian, Karen J., Galina Khatutsky, Thanh V. Tran, and Alan L. Balsam. "Health and Social Service Utilization among Elderly Immigrants from the Former Soviet Union." *Journal of Nursing Scholarship* 33, no. 3 (2001): 265–71.

Benisovich, Sonya V., and Abby C. King. "Meaning and Knowledge of Health among Older Adult Immigrants from Russia: A Phenomenological Study." *Health Education Research* 18, no. 2 (April 2003): 135–44.

Brod, Meryl, and Suzanne Heurtin-Roberts. "Older Russian Emigrés & Medical Care." *The Western Journal of Medicine* special issue, *Cross-Cultural Medicine A Decade Later* 157, no. 3 (September 1992): 333–6.

Duncan, Laura, and Mary Simmons. "Health Practices among Russian and Ukrainian Immigrants." *Journal of Community Health Nursing* 13, no. 2 (1996): 129–37.

Evanikoff, Luba J. "Russians." In *Culture & Nursing Care: A Pocket Guide,* edited by Juliene G. Lipson et al. San Francisco: UCSF Nursing Press, 1996.

Grabbe, Linda. "Understanding Patients from the Former Soviet Union." *Family Medicine* 32, no. 3 (March 2000): 201–6.

Remennick, Larissa. "'I Have No Time for Potential Troubles': Russian Immigrant Women and Breast Cancer Screening in Israel." *Journal of Immigrant Health* 5, no. 4 (October 2003): 153–63.

Smith, Linda. "New Russian Immigrants: Health Problems, Practices & Values." *Journal of Cultural Diversity* 3, no. 3 (Fall 1996): 68–73.

Zander, Kathleen. *Russian Jewish Culture: A Profile in Minnesota.* The Center for Cross-Cultural Health: Minneapolis, 1997.

Chapter 8

Amish

Adams, Carolyn E., and Michael B. Leverland. "The Effects of Religious Beliefs on the Health Care Practices of the Amish." *Nurse Practitioner* 11, no. 3 (March 1986): 58, 63, 67.

Brewer, J. A., and N. M. Bonalumi. "Health Care Beliefs and Practices among the Pennsylvania Amish." *Journal of Emergency Nursing* 21, no. 6 (December 1995): 494–7.

Dellasega, Cheryl, et al. "Culturalizing Health Care for a Culturally Diverse Population: The Amish." *Clinical Excellence for Nurse Practitioners* 3, no. 1 (1999): 10–5.

Fuchs, Janet A., et al. "Health Risk Factors among the Amish: Results of a Survey." *Health Education Quarterly* 17, no. 2 (Summer 1990): 197–211.

Christian Scientists

Gazelle, Gail, Carrie Glover, and Sandra L. Stricklin. "Care of the Christian Science Patient." *Journal of Palliative Medicine* 7, no. 4 (August 2004): 585–8.

Merrick, Janna C. "Spiritual Healing, Sick Kids, and the Law: Inequities in the American Healthcare System." *American Journal of Law & Medicine* 29, nos. 2–3 (2003): 269–99.

Plastine, Laura M. "'In God We Trust': When Parents Refuse Medical Treatment for their Children Based upon Their Sincere Religious Beliefs." *Constitutional Law Journal* 3, no. 1 (Spring 1993): 123–60.

Eastern Orthodox Christians

Davidhizar, Ruth, et al. "Nursing Clients of Greek Ethnicity at Home." *Home Healthcare Nurse* 16, no. 9 (September 1998): 618–23.

Sarri, Katerina O., et al. "Greek Orthodox Fasting Rituals: A Hidden Characteristic of the Mediterranean Diet of Crete." *British Journal of Nutrition* 92, no. 2 (August 2004): 277–84.

Tripp-Reimer, Toni, and Bernard Sorofman. "Greek-Americans." In *Transcultural Health Care: A Culturally Competent Approach* by Larry D. Purnell and Betty J. Paulanka. Philadelphia: F.A. Davis, 1998.

Jehovah's Witnesses

Gyamfi, Cynthia, M.D., Mavis M. Gyamfi, and Richard L. Berkowitz, M.D. "Ethical and MedicolegalConsiderations in the Obstetric Care of a Jehovah's Witness." *Obstetrics & Gynecology* 102, no. 1 (July 2003): 173–80.

Laszlo, Daniele, et al. "Tailored Therapy of Adult Acute Leukaemia in Jehovah's Witnesses: Unjustified Reluctance to Treat." *European Journal of Haematology* 72, no. 4 (April 2004): 264–7.

Nash, Michael J., and Hannah Cohen. "Management of Jehovah's Witness Patients with Haematological Problems." *Blood Reviews* 18, no. 3 (September 2004): 211–7.

Sarteschi, Lelio M. "Jehovah's Witnesses, Blood Transfusions and Transplantations." *Transplantation Procedures* 36, no. 3 (April 2004): 499–501.

Jews

Lewis, Judith A. "Jewish Perspectives on Pregnancy and Childbearing." *American Journal of Maternal and Child Nursing* 28, no. 5 (September/October 2003): 306–12.

Purdy, Sarah, et al. "Demographic Characteristics and Primary Health Care Utilization Patterns of Strictly Orthodox Jewish and Non-Jewish Patients." *Family Practice* 17, no. 3 (June 2000): 233–5.

Selekman, Janice. "Jewish-Americans." In *Transcultural Health Care: A Culturally Competent Approach* by Larry D. Purnell and Betty J. Paulanka. Philadelphia: F.A. Davis, 1998.

Mormons (Church of Jesus Christ of Latter-Day Saints)

Callister, Lynn Clark, Sonia Semenic, and Joyce Cameron Foster. "Cultural and Spiritual Meanings of Childbirth: Orthodox Jewish and Mormon Women." *Journal of Holistic Nursing* 17, no. 3 (September 1999): 280–95.

Conley, L. J., "Childbearing and Childrearing Practices in Mormonism." *Neonatal Network* 9, no. 3 (October 1990): 41–8.

Daniels, Melissa, et al. "Associations between Breast Cancer Risk Factors and Religious Practices in Utah." *Preventive Medicine* 38, no. 1 (January 2004): 28–38.

Rundle, Anne, Maria Carvalho, and Mary Robinson, eds. *Cultural Competence in Health Care: A Practical Guide.* San Francisco: Jossey-Bass, 1999.

Appendix D

Self-Check

The "Developing Cultural Perspective" and "Blending Perspectives" end-of-chapter questions were developed for discussion, and with the exception of a few questions, do not have "right" answers. This answer key can be used as a guide to assist discussion, or can be used as a reference to check for understanding.

CHAPTER ONE

Developing Cultural Perspective

1. Answers may encompass many aspects of popular American culture and will vary depending upon the geographic area of the respondent. Responses to "The Body" questions are likely to encompass a scientific understanding of anatomy. Chronic fatigue syndrome, stress-related disorders, and depression may be listed as examples of a body/mind connection. Answers to "Belief System" questions may incorporate personal beliefs that are not necessarily indicative of general cultural beliefs.

2. Answers will vary depending upon the chapter chosen, answers to chapter 4 may encompass the following:

   Food & Diet: yin/yang balance in food, hot/cold foods, cold foods avoided during illness and after childbirth, avoiding beef and eggs during illness, chicken rice soup for illness, medication taken in liquid forms

   The Body: the head as sacred, blood as a person's essence, blood does not replenish, yin/yang balance in the body, taboo against donating body parts

   Belief System: yin/yang, Qi, Confucianism, gift-giving, Buddhism

3. Answers will vary depending on the cultural background of the person responding. Hopefully, the respondent will take the time to discover similarities as well as differences.

4. Answers should include the following:
   - Speak slowly, not loudly.
   - Face the patient and make extensive use of gestures, pictures, and facial expressions. Watch the patient's face, eyes, and body language carefully.
   - Avoid difficult and uncommon words and idiomatic expressions.
   - Don't "muddy the waters" with unnecessary words or information.
   - Organize what you say for easy access.
   - Rephrase and summarize often.

- Don't ask questions that can be answered by "yes" or "no."
- Check your understanding by paraphrasing what the patient has said.
- Check the concept behind the word.
- Don't burden the patient with decisions he or she is not prepared to make.

Blending Perspectives

1. Common communication elements may include: smiles, crying, frowns, sadness, respect, listening, avoid laughing, beginning on a formal basis, taking time to synthesize and respond, feedback, etc.
2. Elements that **are not** universal among cultures, for example: handshakes, direct eye contact, tone of voice, touch, direct questions, etc. Elements that **are** universal include respect, concern, appreciation, silence, etc.

CHAPTER TWO

Developing Cultural Perspective

1. The belief that treating the symptom does not treat the cause of the disease. The patient may seek a diagnosis from one who looks for the spiritual or emotional connection to the symptom.
2. The normal yellow pigmentation found in dark-skinned individuals tends to be concentrated in the inner and outer canthi of the eyes and in the stool.
3. Absence of red tones.
4. The belief that washing one's hair introduces "cold" to the body. It is believed that "cold" results in illness, and "cold" can clot the blood.
5. Reddish foods such as beets and carrots send an oversupply of blood to the brain and to the heart.
6. Family members may attribute this to a "hex" being placed upon the patient.

Blending Perspectives

1. Answers may discuss the body/mind connection, the traditional separation within Western medical training, and the perspectives from Eastern philosophies that are blending into popular culture.
2. Each respondent will need to find a tone and style that they are comfortable with. They may choose to broaden the question. Examples: "What do you eat to keep your body healthy?" "What do you eat when you are ill?" "Is there any food, liquid, herb, or tonic that you eat or drink that helps you feel better when you are ill?" "Do you consume anything to cleanse your internal organs?"

CHAPTER THREE

Developing Cultural Perspective

1. Extended family play an important part in medical decision and are considered "family." Hospital procedures may limit visitation to the immediate family only. American Indians or Alaska Natives may have a different concept of time and may have difficulty with visitation hours beginning and ending according to a clock.
2. American Indians believe that Mother Earth provides remedies. Explaining the "natural" components of a medication may help it appear more harmonious to their belief system.
3. Avoid prolonged eye contact and do not expect the patient to maintain eye contact, with the exception of an occasional glance to the face.

Blending Perspectives
1. Issues to discuss: the desires of the patient, cultural norms, legal restrictions, consent forms, procedure results, etc.
2. This is a question of human behavior. Response to "tardiness" will vary. Responses may include non-verbal ways of expressing dissatisfaction; body language, curtness, tone of voice, etc.

CHAPTER FOUR

Developing Cultural Perspective
1. They may be unfamiliar with the typical Western diet. They may believe in the importance of balancing yin and yang within the food and that maintaining this balance is important during illness.
2. Typically used to draw out fever and to help restore yin and yang balance, coining, cupping, and moxibustion can leave marks that appear as bruises and discolored spots. The bruises and their placement on the abdomen and forehead could be misinterpreted as abuse.
3. The body must remain "whole," with all its body parts.
4. Hmong believe that each person only has a finite supply of blood and that having blood drawn will make the person weaker and sick.
5. Because of the great importance of the family to Filipinos, the culturally acceptable way to inform a Filipino patient of a negative prognosis or a treatment regimen would be in the presence of a close family member.
6. Ways to ensure that an Asian patient understands the importance of his/her independent treatment regimen include:
   - making sure that the patient completely understands and can repeat back the instructions;
   - using the services of an interpreter;
   - speaking clearly;
   - using simple-but-respectful language;
   - avoiding idiomatic expressions.

Blending Perspectives
1. Discussion may include screening of reports, the rights of patients versus the demands of reporting, protection of children, "innocent until proven guilty," definitions of abuse, assumption of knowledge, etc.
2. Responses may incorporate information from any number of sources that discuss the body/mind connection. They may also include current research, gene theory, genome discoveries, and scientific advances that further the knowledge of the body.
3. Both the ideas of yin and yang and the traditional Asian concepts of "hot" and "cold" are related to balance of substances within the body and in life. In the view of the ideas of yin and yang illness arises from being out of balance. This can be an imbalance of energy or of more tangible aspects of life. One way to restore balance is to ensure that hot aspects are balanced with cold aspects. You could use these concepts to help make your interviews of Asian patients more effective.

CHAPTER FIVE

Developing Cultural Perspective
1. Physical activity is associated with "work," not relaxation.
2. Due to the theory of "hot/cold."
3. A depressed fontanel is viewed as fatal.
4. *Susto*, even though it manifests with physical symptoms, is a spiritual problem.

Blending Perspectives
1. Answers will vary depending on the perspective of the respondent.
2. Discussion may include clinic policy, legal issues, separation of "church and medicine," legal guidelines, ethical guidelines, personal boundary issues, etc.

CHAPTER SIX

Developing Cultural Perspectives
1. Speaking about it may bring it about.
2. They are using their tone to emphasize the importance of what they are saying. You would demonstrate that you were paying attention.
3. They would choose the invasive, believing it to be more effective.
4. Middle Eastern personal boundaries are much closer than what most "Westerners" are used to. It is not uncommon for Middle Easterners to stand very close to each other, and to talk face-to-face.

Blending Perspectives
1. This question asks the respondent to assess his or her personal style.
2. Discussion may include the role of personal responsibility, motivation, "blaming," resignation, etc.

CHAPTER SEVEN

Developing Cultural Perspectives
1. Typical Polish-American diets are high in fat and starch.
2. Medical assistants and nurses are viewed as unskilled and not qualified to make medical decisions.
3. Hospital admissions were quite routine within the Soviet system. Patients may expect to be admitted to a hospital, believing that this is standard procedure and that the quality of care is better than care in a clinic or outpatient setting.
4. There is a stigma against mental health issues. Bosnians may hide these issues and are not comfortable discussing them outside of the family. They may fear that revealing mental health concerns will deny them immigrant status.
5. Answers will vary but may include sharing information about training, case studies, testimonials, etc.
6. A Bosnian patient might be especially frustrated and angry at having to wait an hour-and-a-half to see a Western doctor because in Bosnia he or she probably would not have had to wait at all. Medical procedures that are completed by Western highly trained nurses and nurse practitioners might be viewed as not as good as the same procedures done by physicians. A Bosnian patient also might think that U.S. hospitals and physicians do not provide enough attention and care to their patients and might view them as for-profit organizations.

CHAPTER EIGHT

Developing Cultural Perspectives

1. You should be wary of praising infants and young children in front of their parents because the parents might see it as drawing the evil eye or causing bad luck.

2. You could maximize the success of your interactions with and treatments for an Old Order Amish patient by using the following strategies:
   - try to build trust with the patient by showing that you appreciate their unique cultural ways;
   - rely more heavily on your clinical skills and judgment and less on diagnostic tests that may be unnecessary;
   - thoroughly explain the need for treatments to patients, caregivers, and/or authority figures.

3. Standard hospital procedures that might be upsetting include:
   - to a faithful Mormon: requirement to remove the traditional undergarment
   - an Orthodox Jew: requiring a woman to remove a wig or head covering
   - a Sikh: requiring removal of turban or cutting hair

4. An Old Order Amish patient might delay medical treatment because it is inconvenient to travel or because the patient has been trying herbal or other traditional remedies and waiting for the condition to improve.

5. Christian Scientists view illness as a sign that prayer is needed to reestablish harmony in all aspects of a person's life. When harmony is reestablished, healing will proceed. Christian Scientists will reject any medical treatment that goes against their religious beliefs, including medications and surgery.

Blending Perspectives

1. Answers to these questions will vary widely, depending upon personal beliefs and opinions.

2. Answers should analyze interactions with patients and especially look for instances where the practitioner was either condescending or expressed self-importance. Answers to the second part of the question will vary, but realizing that other people's religion is at least as important to them as yours is to you, is one way to begin to improve and change your style of interacting with diverse patients and their families to foster their trust.